COME,
LET ME
GUIDE YOU

New Directions in the Human-Animal Bond
Alan M. Beck and Marguerite E. O'Haire, series editors

COME, LET ME GUIDE YOU

A Life Shared
with a Guide Dog

Susan Krieger

Purdue University Press
West Lafayette, Indiana

Printed in the United States of America.

Library of Congress Cataloging-in-Publication Data

Krieger, Susan.
  Come, let me guide you : a life shared with a guide dog / Susan Krieger.
      pages cm. -- (New directions in the human-animal bond)
  Includes bibliographical references.
  ISBN 978-1-55753-714-0 (hardback : alk. paper) -- ISBN 978-1-61249-389-3 (epdf) -- ISBN 978-1-61249-390-9 (epub)
1. Krieger, Susan. 2. Guide dogs--United States--Biography.
3. Blind--United States--Biography. 4. Human-animal
relationships--United States. I. Title.
  HV1780.K75 2015
  362.4'1092--dc23
  [B]
                              2015014481

To obtain an accessible version of this book, please contact the
publisher at pupress@purdue.edu.

Cover photo courtesy of Estelle Freedman.

For Estelle

Contents

Preface

THE JOURNEY THAT BEGAN when I first came home with Teela has taken me through loss of vision, deaths of dear ones, and an increased intimacy with my partner; it has taken me through playful times on grassy fields as I happily tossed a Frisbee to Teela; and it has made me feel more welcome in the world than I ever was before—because people now greeted me with the pleasure of also meeting my dog.

I want to thank the staff of Guide Dogs for the Blind for breeding, training, and nurturing Teela and for their support of both of us as a pair. I am indebted to Teela's "puppy raisers"—Betsy, Galen, Emily, and Spencer McCray—who cared for and socialized this lively, loving dog during her first sixteen months. Jim Power, our Guide Dogs field representative, visited Teela and me each year after our graduation to check on our well-being, providing expert instruction and support. When the time came for Teela to retire, Jim trained me with a second guide dog, Fresco, easing the transition. I am grateful to Fresco's puppy raisers—Patty, Mike, and Klamath Henry—who gave him such a good start in life.

Most of all, I am indebted to Estelle Freedman, my intimate partner, who has guided me often when I have lost a sense of direction. For over three decades, Estelle has been a joy and an inspiration for me who has helped make all else possible. She improved each draft of *Come, Let Me Guide You*, knowing, more than anyone else, the importance of my conveying an inner sense of reality and the nuances of the life I have shared with Teela. In this book, I refer to Estelle as "Hannah" to indicate that this is but my version of our shared experience.

My second closest reader of these stories has been Paola Gianturco, who encouraged the intimacy of my writing and provided invaluable editorial advice. To the extent that *Come, Let Me Guide You* is clear, expressive of feeling, and conveys a sense of inner freedom, it is because, as I wrote it, I often was guided by the thought, "I think Paola will like this." Everyone should have such a superb muse.

During the six years while I was writing this book, treasured friends and colleagues gave me helpful input on specific chapters and the organization of the whole. I would like especially to thank: Susan Cahn, Zandra Contaxis, Lynn Crawford, Carmen de Monteflores, Hal Kahn, and Ilene Levitt. Angelica Bammer and Ruth-Ellen Boetcher Joeres helped shape "The Art of the Intimate Narrative" when it was originally prepared as an outgrowth of a conference on "How We Write: Scholarly Writing and the Power of Form." Martin Krieger generously offered encouragement and contributed the chapter title "A New Pair of Eyes." I thank my sister, Kathe Morse, both for her insights on chapters and for helping me with the challenging task of representing our mother in "My Mother's Bracelet." Susan Christopher closely read the entire manuscript, polishing my prose, clarifying where needed, and suggesting improvements to the flow of the whole. I thank her for her keen editorial eye, her good sense, and her ability to suggest changes in keeping with my poetic style.

At Purdue University Press, Director Charles Watkinson and Series Editor Alan Beck were graciously receptive to the idea of this book and then helpfully encouraging of my efforts both to tell a specific story of my life with Teela and to make a broader contribution. I thank Katherine Purple for her generosity, her sensitive copyediting, and her tasteful book design; Bryan Shaffer for production and marketing and for the beautiful cover design, done in collaboration with Heidi Branham; and Rebecca Corbin for valuable administrative assistance. Shelley Fisher Fishkin and Esther Rothblum critically reviewed the manuscript, providing insightful comments and suggestions.

Because *Come, Let Me Guide You* draws on experiences I have shared with others, I wish to thank all those who have made the moments I describe here especially meaningful for me. They may appear in my stories under pseudonyms or anonymously, but they have supported my explorations and have figured more largely in my inner life than a brief mention might suggest. I thank the students in my Women and Disabilities seminar at Stanford University during 2002–2014 for contributing to my learning about disabilities and for welcoming Teela into our classroom. I am particularly grateful to Jessi Aaron, Audrey Dufrechou, Maja Falcon, Julia Feinberg, Rasha Glenn, Amelia Herrera, Shayla Parker, and Tania Tran.

I thank Phoebe Wood for directing me to the San Pedro Cemetery the year my mother died, where I found the grave of another "beloved mother," Francisca Saavedra, and a way to help deal with my loss. I am grateful to my uncle, Herbert Lewis, for his memories of my mother, and to my sister and her family—Kathe, Rich, Rachel, Julia, and Beth Morse—with whom I shared the experience of my mother's last days and the honoring of her memory. I thank my mother, Rhoda Cahn, in memoriam, for the love of life she passed on to me and for being smart, caring, and all-knowing. I continue to be indebted to Carolyn Hallowell for eighteen years of constancy and for being with me still, her legacy now carried on by two beautiful golden guide dogs.

Louise Sholes wrote the original poem from which this book gains its title. I was deeply moved when I heard it read aloud at Teela's Guide Dogs for the Blind graduation ceremony in October 2003, and it has been an inspiration for me ever since. I also thank Klamath Henry for her moving words read at Fresco's Guide Dogs graduation in October 2013, and quoted in the book's closing chapter. I am indebted, of course, to Teela and to Fresco, who have helped me learn to trust, moved me through the world with speed and ease, and enabled me to feel less alone.

Estelle Freedman has been with me through all the experiences described in this book. As I follow Teela through these stories, holding tightly to the harness handle, Estelle is always by my side—watching out for us, protecting us, leading at times, following at others, urging me forward, making sure no obstacle ahead is insurmountable. She has welcomed two guide dogs into our life with the same generosity as she has long welcomed me into hers. I thank her with all my heart.

Introduction

For over a decade, I have had the privilege of sharing my life with a guide dog, a Golden Retriever-yellow Labrador named Teela. During this period, the relationship between us has changed both of our lives. This is a book about being led by a dog to new places in the world and new places in myself, a book about facing life's challenges outwardly and within, and about reading those clues—those deeply felt signals—that can help guide the way. It is also, more broadly, about the importance of intimate connection in human-animal relationships, academic work, and personal life. It is about the company we keep, about companionship, guidance, interdependence, and love.

In these stories, I describe how my relationship with Teela has had far-reaching effects—influencing not only my abilities to navigate the world while blind, but my writing, my teaching, and my sense of self. I explore my inner emotions as I walk with her, no longer facing the world alone but accompanied by her spirited presence, and I examine other intimate relationships in my life that have been enriched and supported by our bond. Yet these reflections are more than strictly personal. Throughout, I draw insights from my experiences that I hope may prove helpful to others—guide dog and service dog users, individuals with pets or those who also share their lives with animals, and readers interested in issues of intimacy and interconnectedness more generally. For, as these stories suggest, a relationship with a guide dog has much in common with other intimate connections, and the search for self that it encourages is akin to other individual quests for competence, comfort, and self-worth.

In my previous book, *Traveling Blind: Adventures in Vision with a Guide Dog by My Side*, I explored my first two years with Teela as we traveled city streets and country byways and as I learned to perceive the world in new ways. As I wrestled with dilemmas of self-acceptance and dealt with how I was perceived by others, I grew to appreciate my own particular ways of seeing, even if limited, and to value my blindness as well as my sight. In that book, our relationship was just beginning to form. *Come, Let Me Guide You* extends the narrative as I follow Teela through the entire ten-year span of our working life together. Here I describe how the intimacy between us developed in intensity and naturalness over time and how, as Teela led me around external obstacles, she was also leading me around inner ones, enabling me to confront life's complexities with a newfound freedom. The book chronicles the exhilaration of our early years, the deepening of our relationship during our middle period, and the enduring intimacy of our bond. The chapters are organized in topical groupings pertinent to our journey. At the end of each, I give the date it was originally written to help the reader navigate the chronology.

Part I, "Sharing the Road," provides a detailed account of what life has been like for us over the years—beginning with Teela's older age as I face the prospect of her imminent retirement. I then look back on our earlier times, exploring significant moments from when she was young. In walking with her, I discover new pleasures, adapting my life to hers as she does to mine. I learn to read her signals as she guides me and to reflect on my own inner responses—the feelings of profound gratitude and joy she raises in me. These chapters convey Teela's lively yet deferential temperament. At one moment, she will seem to be a "party girl"—eager to play and have a good time—and, at the next, she is my "dutiful guide"—stopping at curbs, leading me around dangers and through dark or difficult times, turning toward me often to make sure I am still following her. Her outgoing personality clearly complements my more introverted nature and enhances my abilities both to contribute to others and to face challenges within myself.

In Part II, "Searching for Sight," I focus on my blindness and my struggles for sight, which continue to be a challenge for me even with Teela's guidance. Here I share with the reader the experience of facing javelinas in the Chiricahua mountains of Arizona, seeking to protect my curious guide dog from small tusked animals I cannot see; the adventure of going shopping for a camera with Teela by my side as I try to use this equipment for the sighted to reach beyond the limits of my blindness; and our travels in the New Mexico desert, where I confront the peculiar fact that although I can look up and see large white clouds in a bright blue sky, I cannot see the ground at my feet and I often fear that I will stumble and fall even as Teela guides me. In this section, traveling with Teela provides entrée into a broader discussion of dilemmas of vision and blindness.

In Part III, "Weathering Life's Losses," I draw from our middle years, branching out to examine other intimate relationships in my life that, like my tie with Teela, have prompted insight and self-reflection. In these stories, Teela is often an invisible partner, but her companionship is vital to my equilibrium—as I visit my mother's bedside in the days before she died; as I stand in a distant cemetery, thinking back on my life with this challenging woman who raised me; when I visit my sister to go through my mother's jewelry; and then as I wear my mother's silver Navajo bracelet to remind me of positive qualities she has passed down to me. Teela's importance to my inner life is further explained in the subsequent chapter as I confront the loss of a psychotherapist who guided me emotionally for eighteen years. I remember how, as I walked to my therapist's memorial service, probing ahead of me with my white cane, I imagined having a golden dog who would carry her spirit and be always by my side. Not long afterward, I got Teela, who soon became an extension of that important bond. In a concluding chapter, I describe how having Teela with me, and thus always the possibility of our taking off on an energetic walk, has imbued my life with a sense of openness to adventure that has helped me through the self-doubt that followed upon these two intimate losses.

In Part IV, "Seeking Connection," I explain my "intimate narrative" approach to ethnography and discuss the influence of my relationship with Teela on my academic work. I describe how she has figured in my research and writing much as she has in my personal life—an external presence that has enabled me to explore my sense of myself and to become more at home in the world. In the subsequent chapter, I draw from my experiences teaching a life-altering course on women and disabilities at Stanford University, where Teela lay under the seminar table, contributing to the comfort of the classroom and to my confidence as a teacher. It was in that course, the first year I taught it, that a student had appeared with a guide dog, making me wish the same for myself, although at that time I was only starting to use a white cane.

The connections between past and present merge in the concluding chapter as I describe my joy and Teela's playful cooperation when I receive a new guide dog named Fresco and as both Teela and I seek to get to know him and to school him in our ways. As I walk with Fresco, I keep Teela always in my mind, guiding me on how to be in the world, how to share my pleasures and face new experiences with confidence. I miss her and yet I am determined not to leave her behind. The themes of the book concerning intimacy, self-reflection, and needs for external support for inner identity echo through this last chapter on life with two guide dogs—one retired but still leading me in spirit, and the other newly guiding me, causing me, as Teela did, to reflect on my inner life as well as on the outer paths we explore.

Because each of these stories was written with a different main focal point—each examining a different type of intimate experience—Teela's presence is central and explicit in some of them, while in others, it is often implicit. She is an invisible companion by my side, as guide dogs typically are for their users, yet she is no less important when unseen. A second often invisible presence in these pages is that of Hannah, my human partner for the past thirty-four years, who welcomed Teela into our life and who has helped care for and guide both of us. Her loving companionship has deeply informed the openness and honesty of these stories.

Come, Let Me Guide You extends the personal approach of my prior studies, beginning with *Social Science and the Self: Personal Essays on an Art Form* (1991), in which I argued for a more full use of the subjectivity of an observer in social research. Over time, my ethnographic narratives have become increasingly intimate, and *Come, Let Me Guide You* takes a step forward in this approach by speaking emotionally and from the heart. At the same time, the book is intended as a contribution to the academic field of human-animal studies, offering insights about human-animal communication and a detailed exploration of changes that occur over the life span of a working pair. It is further intended as a contribution to disability studies, feminist studies, and sociological methodology, elaborating understandings of personal identity and expanding possibilities for representation through the use of personal narrative. Its place in the literature of each of these fields is detailed in the Bibliographic Notes.

This book was written during 2008–2014, over a period of nearly six years when I was increasingly, though gradually, losing my eyesight to a condition called "birdshot retinochoroidopathy." This is an autoimmune disease that has caused inflammation and scarring on my retina and that I have had since 1996. It has resulted in blind areas throughout my central and peripheral vision, increased darkness, blurring, color loss, distortion, lack of depth perception, and inability to see fine lines and details. Often I will see the shape of something directly in front of me, but I will miss an object one inch to the side. I am constantly trying to figure out what I see, because I see it only partially, and soon it may disappear. Mine is an irregular type of vision, a spotty blindness that comes and goes, sometimes fading into the background, sometimes calling my attention to it, such as when I stumble or fall or hit my head on an open door because I do not see it, or when I lose my way, even in a familiar area, because the shapes and forms around me seem indistinct, the paths between them unclear.

Yet amidst all the uncertainty of what I see and seek to know, there has been, for the past ten years, a large golden dog by my side, usually a few steps ahead guiding me into the future. Far more than an aid to my blindness, she has been an aid to my sense of self—providing me with an external footing, a third leg on the tripod, a self outside myself to whom others say, "What a beautiful dog," or, "Tell me her name," so that when with her, I walk through the world far less anonymously than I ever expected to be and with a sureness and sense of pride that I would not have on my own. A further benefit of life with Teela has been that she has always loved to play. For ten years, I have carried a floppy Frisbee in my backpack that comes out when we are on a college campus, or visiting my mother, or at home but in need of exercise or escape. I toss it to Teela and she returns it to me, bounding off and coming back with great glee—her spirit, her openness to adventure and joy, enhancing and causing reflection on my own. In these stories, I attempt to convey a sense of our relationship and how the intimacy it has provided for me has been intertwined with so many other aspects of my life. I hope that my insights and sharing of experiences may prove fruitful for the reader, encouraging a sense of new direction or knowledge, or simply a familiarity with what life has been like for me. Come, let me guide you.

Part I

Sharing the Road

ONE

+ ✦✦✦ +

An Older Guide Dog

MY GUIDE DOG, TEELA, is eleven now. I have had her since she was twenty-two months old. She was a big golden puppy then. She still has that same liveliness, although she is now a much lighter shade of gold, with many white hairs mixed in with her blond. I take her for granted much of the time, because she is always by my side. Sometimes she is in another room basking in the sunlight while I am at my computer. But most of the time she is with me, no more than an arm's length away. Our relationship has changed over the years. I think we have become more attuned to each other, more intricately connected. That seems natural for a relationship over time, but it always surprises me. She knows when she hears the zipper as I take out my backpack that I am getting ready to go out with her. She knows that when I whisper a command to her—"Sit," "Stay," "Lie down now"—that I am deadly serious, and she obeys the whisper when she will not obey a loud or harsh command. I think perhaps the loud command jars her, frightens her, or puts her off. The whisper is reassuring. It's a direct communication from me to her—a statement of our intimacy.

I am sad as I start to review my relationship with Teela, and I feel that I should not be sad. Because Teela is still with me, still guiding me, even though we both know she is ready for retirement and has been now for about a year. But the guide dog organization has not found a suitable replacement dog for me yet, and I have insisted on receiving the right dog—as if Teela has spoiled me, made me feel that only another like her will meet my needs. She has formed those needs, taught me with her interactions with me where I can go, how to take my steps, how to process those moments in between getting from here to there when we simply occupy space together—how to reach out to her with my feelings, respond to her, to a look in her face, the feel of her brow, her fur, her eager excitement, her readiness for my next step. Much of the day, I am relating to this dog, to her temperament, her presence. I know, all the time, where she is. I think of her needs as I do my own, almost in the same breath. Will Teela want to go to the restaurant? Will she be comfortable there? Will she lick the floor? Would she like a long walk right now? Is her dinner going to be too late on the day when I am working on campus? Will I need to bring along her food? Will she want to stop at the bank where they have dog treats? When we go to the desert wildlife refuge, will she be cold in the back of the car when I get out with my camera and telephoto lens to try to see the birds rising at dawn? Will she be glad when we get to the desert? Will it seem worth the uncomfortable plane ride full of vibrations and noises that so distress her? Does she like the desert as much as I do? Will she ever forgive me for not letting her chase cats, and rabbits, and stray balls that roll down the street on the hill in front of our house?

Teela is a retriever at heart. If I offer her food in one hand and her floppy Frisbee in the other, she will take the Frisbee. Being a guide dog is second nature to her; her first nature is retrieving, and I have taken that into account, built that into the way we live together—so that always she can retrieve. When we travel and are in the country, I can throw her floppy Frisbee to her every day. We have been through many Frisbees over the years, using them until they are full of holes from her catching them in mid-air with her sharp teeth, bringing them back, shaking them at me, and asking that I throw to her again. In the basement of my house, I have, at any one time, several sturdy, almost indestructible, toys that Teela retrieves daily, carrying them gleefully up the back stairs, dropping them just outside the kitchen door—there for me to pick up from the floor so I do not trip on them. Then I take them downstairs later so that she can retrieve them again. She is gleeful about retrieving, dutiful about guiding, happy to meet people when she is not working—when she is "off harness." Often she is still working when out of her harness, but at other times she is free. She knows from how I talk to her whether she is working or not. We communicate in ways we have learned. I say "okay" to release her, give a nod of my head and a pat on her back, a command to go greet a person, and then she wiggles and wags all she wants, though always she looks back over at me—more attuned than the usual dog to exactly what I will expect of her next.

I carry her harness, at times, when we walk and she is not wearing it, which is to say, I often wear the harness—slung over my left shoulder. This makes me feel that I am relieving her of some of the burden. I feel, all the more, that we are in this together, and a bit like what she may feel when she wears it. When we go to the beach, I take the harness off her and walk with her beside me, not guiding me, but heeling on the leash. Or I attempt to get her to heel. She really wants to guide, to lead, even when the harness is off. I try to keep her beside me, but she gets ahead, still taking me, taking me everywhere. She expects me to share her exuberance for the waves, the next piece of seaweed, the smell of a rock or piece of driftwood. All that her nose touches she finds positively fascinating.

Given the great enjoyment of life that she brings me, why am I so sad? Because I know Teela is going to retire soon, and though I will keep her, I fear losing her. It feels, in advance, as if she will die. She likely has years left. She is a healthy dog and can live to about fifteen. But her upcoming retirement feels like a small death, mine perhaps as well as hers—a loss of all the ways I have learned to be blind with her, the ways I have integrated my blindness with who I am. For Teela represents not only my sight, but my acceptability in the world. When I walk with her, I walk with pride. It is hard to imagine no longer doing so. I feel, too, that I will be letting her down. I can see now that look that will come to her eyes—you are going out without me, why?

When I first got Teela, I kept trying to push out of my mind the fact that she would eventually have to retire. At a certain point, guide work would become too much of a strain for her. They told us at guide dog school that each of our dogs had a "puppy raiser" during their first sixteen months, and that eventually someone would take them when they were ready to retire, or we or a family member could keep our dog. I never expected that I would be keeping Teela. I felt, how could I manage with another pet dog, and three cats, and a not very large house in the city? The prospect of Teela's retirement was always the prospect of losing her to someone else, and I worried about whether they would take care of her well enough, and how she would survive if she missed me. Now, even though my partner, Hannah, and I will happily be keeping her, Teela's retirement remains an event overshadowed with loss. I expect that when I get a new guide dog, I will feel differently. Because the new guide—or at least this was so in Teela's case—will bring me new life, a new excitement, a new sense of adventure. When I get the new dog, I may not feel the loss of Teela as much, and Teela will be happy in retirement, too, I think. She is an upbeat, lively, cheerful dog. But now she seems ready to have more rest.

She still takes pleasure in doing her work—guiding me in the open air, in and out of buildings and stores, going to the university campus, greeting people, coming with me almost everywhere. But the physical work takes a lot out of her, far more than it used to. She is more reliant on small non-guidework pleasures—the treat at the bank, the times when she will run free and chase her Frisbee, the quiet comforts of her home.

For over a year, Teela has been giving me hints that the world is more bothersome to her than it once was, and that she needs a greater sense of protection than guide dogs usually require. When we walk down the street, if there is construction noise ahead, instead of leading me safely past it, she now stops, not wanting to go on. She stares up at me. I give her a command to go forward, but she will not budge. She then turns us around and leads back to the previous corner, where we cross to the other side of the street and continue in our original direction, but farther from the noise. I sometimes try to coax her so that she will not turn back. I stand beside her, pat her head, and talk to her, explaining that the construction noises will not hurt her. I give her leash one more strong yank forward to indicate we should move ahead. But increasingly, I wish not to argue with her when she has decided something is not safe. I feel she is older now and that she deserves my honoring her choices.

Occasionally we face a more serious quandary. Not long ago, I was in downtown San Francisco for an appointment at the dentist. I was early and Teela and I were walking the streets for our exercise. As we turned one busy corner and started up the street, I heard huge construction noises mid-block—abrasive machines, drills cutting up the cement, generator motors. People were walking on a narrow pathway within the street at the edge of it. I could not see well enough to know exactly how they got there, or if the sidewalk had a clearing. The noise was deafening and Teela put on her brakes. "Forward," I told her, urging her on, but she would not go. I stepped up beside her head, gave a more firm command and a tug, and leaned my body into it to indicate this was serious, there was no time for fear now, "Just get us out of here." But no Teela movement. She stood her ground, looked back at me, and started to back up. There was no way we would be going forward past the construction. To go back down the street would mean traveling a long way around through many oddly angled streets, which I did not want to do. Here

I was, overwhelmed by the noise myself, unable to discern a path, with a frozen dog beside me—rightfully frozen, but frozen nonetheless—who would neither lead me to the pathway in the street where other people were walking nor proceed on the sidewalk.

I decided I had no other choice but to ask the construction crew to turn off their machines. I was about to do so when a worker close to me approached. He offered his arm and indicated, with a broad gesture of his hands, that it was all right for us to pass near their equipment. But Teela would have none of it. Then, fortunately, a pedestrian, who was walking up the narrow passageway in the street, came over to us and offered that we follow him. Somehow that was reassuring enough for Teela, who took a cue from me and turned left, and then we ran up that street—past the machinery, past the other pedestrians hugging the edge of the narrow walkway. Never again would I put her through that, I thought. I would walk the long way around next time. I did not like her being so scared. Yet sometimes it is unavoidable. Teela is afraid of so much now, though perhaps not always afraid as much as she is cautious, careful, and self-protective. If there is some possible adverse consequence that will follow from a loud noise or a threat, she does not want to find that out. She is a guide dog even in her older age. She has long watched out for our safety, and now will do no less. If she fears for herself or feels she needs to proceed with extra care, then I, attached by the bond of the harness, follow her, figuring it out on the run.

In the past year, Teela has sought to avoid buses as well as construction. When we walk by a bus stop and a bus approaches, with its loud engine noises and hissing air brakes, she starts to run to get away from it. At one particularly busy bus stop on a local commercial street that she knows from the past, she bolts as soon as we get near it. She breaks into a gallop, with me in tow, racing past the stop to let me know that she does not want to get on a bus. It is an uphill walk to our house and we may be tired, but I walk it with her. Her needs are so clear. She would rather exert the extra effort for the climb than take that noisy mode of transport, and she then walks briskly and cheerfully, delighted with her new freedom.

At those times when we do board a bus, the internal noises discomfort her—even those of the electric buses—their vibrations and rattling, the closed internal space, the jostling about up and down on the hills. We enter and Teela quickly sits at my feet, where I prop her up between my legs to steady and protect her. I pat her head and hold her close, grasping the top strap of her harness to help keep her upright when the bus lurches. If there are prolonged loud clanks and hisses or big vibrations, she starts to shed; her hair goes flying. I know this although I cannot see it. I can feel her shake. People say to me, "What a beautiful dog," but I know I have a frightened dog who cannot wait to rush off the bus. And when our stop comes, she bolts, carrying me quickly down the stairs and out the front door, where we both catch our breath, sigh with relief, and feel pleased to be out again in the open air where Teela can guide, not be cooped up, not be frightened. I look forward to when I will no longer have to take Teela on buses. We do it rarely now and she is adapted to a few short rides a week, but she reminds me every time, as she seeks to run past the stop, that this is not for her. It is something she does, when needed, for me.

My guide's greater cautiousness extends to her indoor life as well. She often waits for a long time at a door before entering a room. In the house, when we come up from the basement, she waits at the back door to the kitchen, as if wanting to make sure that no cat is on the other side who will leap up at her, though our cats have never done that. If I open the kitchen door just a crack, then give her permission to enter, thinking she will push the door open farther and walk in, she continues to wait—until I pick up on her cue and push the door open fully so that she can have a wider view. Happily, then, she steps inside, with me following, feeling I am slow to adapt to her needs but that I am glad to make the world feel safer for her. As I witness her greater self-protectiveness, it is a lesson to me. This is something she does because she is older. It is all right and to be respected.

Teela clearly tires more easily now. After a walk of a few blocks, she breathes harder than she used to. If I walk with her late in the day, she will be slower than in the past, and she will be more tired on the return and may drag her right back leg. This is why I sometimes take the bus back with her when we do errands on a commercial street that is far enough away that it will tax her. If I go out with her early in the morning, she has more energy for the return. I sometimes take her on Saturday morning to a farmer's market, where she eagerly finds pieces of carrots and vegetables that have fallen to the ground, then walks the full way back without stress. I am careful not to overdo things with her, not to make her walks too long, her exercise periods too strenuous. I have always been careful. Since she was young, I have wanted not to have her injure her knees or her legs; I have wanted to avoid anything that might impede her ability to guide me. I have given her plenty of exercise to keep her muscles in shape. I continue to do so now, but I have to be more careful about her vulnerabilities.

I can't throw the Frisbee high in the air to her anymore. If she reaches up too far forward to catch it, she may strain her upper back. She has already done that and is now recovering. So I throw the Frisbee low and she chases it, scoops it up from the ground. We play on the university campus on the big expanses of manicured grass on those days I am teaching. We play on the beach in the sand, but not for too long because running in soft sand is a strain for a dog. We play as we used to—simply not as strenuously—so that Teela will have her pleasures but not hurt herself. As I adjust our activities, I am acutely aware that my golden girl is getting older. This makes her seem all the more precious to me.

On airplanes, Teela has become more nervous. She sheds her fur furiously when the plane takes off. She has always done this, but, in recent years, she sheds more and has become reluctant to lie down at my feet where we sit in the bulkhead section. The vibrations coming up through the floor and the noises from the plane's engine seem like threats to her. She tries to stand and to circle in place and will do so for hours. I work with her to calm her down. I stroke her back as we take off, holding her close, making her sit. I attempt to settle her afterward, putting my head down low near hers, talking to her, taking her harness off, pushing her rear end down, trying to shift her body weight to make her lie at my feet. She will sit or lie down for a minute, then get up and try to circle again. The only thing that truly works is when she eventually finds a position where she can lie with her body stretched out at my feet, but with her nose out in the aisle, looking toward the door and the activities of the flight attendants. During the flight, she gradually edges farther into the aisle so that eventually her entire head is out. I imagine passengers farther back with clear views of the head of my dog. I repeatedly pull her in toward me, and then she will put her head out again. Usually the flight attendants, very considerately, step over her, though when the refreshment cart comes up the aisle, they alert me and I retract my dog. As I leave the plane, the passengers tell me what a well-behaved dog she was, and I wonder, didn't they see her head? But she has been well behaved. She has lain still, stretched out, found a way to be comfortable with where I have to go, abided my constant attempts to settle her, accompanied me on yet another airplane trip, long past the time when she could better tolerate it. When the plane lands and we get off, she is the first one out, speeding up the ramp, carrying me with her to our freedom.

Because of the stresses involved, I have not taken long plane rides in the past year, only a short flight to New Mexico. On our last trip there this past December, Teela enjoyed playing in the snow, the privacy of being with Hannah and me on this special getaway, the smells and wildlife of the desert, the comforts of home in the places we stayed, the everyday experience of chasing her Frisbee. Yet there clearly were times when she spoke to me through her fears—when the noisy heater in the rental house clattered, when she was tired of jumping up into the car, a small SUV that was higher from the ground than a sedan, and I had to lure her in with a treat. But at no time were her cautions more pronounced than in the rental car parking lot on our return.

We were leaving the car off and had unloaded our bags and checked the interior for anything remaining. The car was empty, but for Teela. She sat on the back seat, with the door open, looking out. I reached in and attached her leash to her collar, a signal to her that it is time to jump down. But she just sat there, brakes on. I heard faint sounds of airplanes overhead in the distance and thought she was afraid of getting on a plane. I gave her leash a firm tug and told her, "Down." She stood on the seat then—a tall golden statue. I unbuckled her harness and took it off, knowing that sometimes she will not want to get in or out of a car when she anticipates that her harness might get caught on a door, the car ceiling, or a front seat—when she feels there is not enough space for both her and it. But no movement occurred. I may have resorted to offering her a treat, though it is not something I usually do in that circumstance. Finally, she gave in and jumped down out of the car, and off we went.

Only as we approached the car rental building did I find out the root of her problem. Huge buses were pulling up to the curb in front of the building to shuttle people to and from the airline terminal. These were very noisy buses, and even from the distance of the car in the parking lot, Teela could hear them, and she paid attention to them, when I did not. As we stepped up onto the sidewalk, seeing the buses so close, she stopped, with a finality that shocked me. I patted her head, ran my hand down her back, and felt the rigidity of her stance. This wasn't going to be easy. I gave her the command to go forward. She refused. I started to coax. "We have to get on it," I said. "We don't. I can't," she responded. "I am a dog. I am your nearly retired guide. I don't like buses anymore. I never did. They sound awful. You wouldn't if you were a dog. You wouldn't if you were me. I may look big and golden, like a cuddly bear. I may look like I can take anything, like my good nature is ever expanding. But I am older now. I don't like these things. Help me."

After some wheedling and pulling, we got on the bus. We made it home. But I look forward to the day when I don't have to put Teela through these barrages of distressing stimuli—even though I dread no longer having her with me, no longer having our back-and-forth conversations. At those times when Teela has put on her brakes, she always furrows her brow as we speak—as if letting me know that only a certain amount of our talking together will get her to understand that I have taken her complaints seriously—that I know how she feels, and though we need to go on, I will protect her, keep her with me, not let any dreadful wrongness befall her.

I imagine that one day I will be traveling with another guide dog who is not as afraid or as uncomfortable on airplanes. It's hard to imagine another dog, not Teela. And yet I do think of it. Sometimes that other dog is her opposite—a tall black male. I find it easier to imagine her opposite than another dog very like her. That feels too confusing, though probably it would be a good idea for me. I am so attached to her.

When we come home from outings that have had distressing noises in them—or been tiring, or led us far away—Teela will often immediately get in one of the small dog beds we have in the house that I originally bought for our black miniature poodle, Esperanza. These beds are oval-shaped, made of foam, and lined with fleece. They are just the size for Teela if she makes herself as compact as possible and curls up in a ball. The padded sides of the bed then envelop her, as if someone is holding her. There she feels protection. She is happy, head tucked beneath her tail, a gold mass almost overflowing the bed. Hannah and I sit at the dining table and remark, "Big dog in small bed. Little dog in big bed"—seeing Esperanza's black shape in the much larger bed that should be Teela's.

Recently when there are loud construction noises outside, Teela will get under Hannah's desk in the house, away from windows, or she'll stay down in the basement in her favorite bed—the bed I gave her when she first arrived home nine and-a-half years ago. I fed her next to it, separately from our other animals, so she and I could continue to bond as I taught her, over and over, her place. Though home with me, she was still a guide dog, different from others, stepping to her own schedule, to the ways of being we had learned in our training so that we could move through the world as a pair.

From the start when I came home with her, Hannah and I would occasionally refer to Teela as our "simple girl." Her needs and wants were clear—in comparison, that is, to Esperanza, who is always trying to get her way, to figure us out, possibly outsmart us, definitely behaving like an alpha dog. Teela is more deferential, more a middle child. Over time, however, I think that Teela has become more complex as a result of our many interactions. And being more complex, she is harder for me to lose. I sense more depth, more sensitivity, more subtle attentiveness on her part, more self-expression in her responsiveness to me. Still I know she remains, in many ways, that original simple girl—happy to retrieve, happy to curl up in her bed, happy to find the next smell, to walk beside me, to guide me, to eat, to reach the bank for her treat, to wag and wiggle excitedly upon greeting a new person.

During the past year while I have been waiting for a new guide and sharing with Teela the stresses she experiences, I have come to value her in her older age. I have come to value her cautions and hesitations, her being not a different dog so much as a more self-protective one. This period of our interrelatedness has made it even harder for me to feel that she and her temperament will not always be with me as I walk the streets, take my plane flights. I may be able to walk for longer, travel farther, not worry as much about my dog when I get my next guide. But where will Teela be? She will be in my mind all the time as I compare the new dog to her, I am sure. I did not always have this depth of feeling regarding Teela. When she was more robust and could do seemingly anything, when she was more indifferent to loud noises and potential threats, I was less aware of her sensitivities. The complexities of my dog were hidden, not as apparent to me. Experiencing her in her older age—though it is not old age so much as her older-than-working age—has given me a great appreciation for this time of her life, the specialness of it. I feel it is a privilege to keep company with her, and I value her more than I ever did. I feel, too, that the advantages of a younger dog are far outweighed by the sensitivities of sharing life with the older one. Yet Teela is a continuity. As we walk, I also walk with the younger Teela, the dog I first came home with nine and-a-half years ago.

April 2013

TWO

When She Was Young

TEELA WAS BORN AT GUIDE DOGS for the Blind in San Rafael, California, in November 2003, one of a litter of ten puppies, seven of whom graduated from guide dog training to be placed with a blind user. Her father was a Labrador Retriever, reddish-blond in color, her mother a red-blond Golden Retriever. Teela is tall—a Golden Retriever-Labrador cross with short, strawberry blond fur, lively in temperament from the start. Her first eight weeks were spent in the guide dog puppy enclosures, where she was with her littermates and intensively socialized with people and objects of the world with which she would need to be familiar.

A family in Weaverville, California, raised her for her next fourteen months. She was initially a 4-H project of the daughter's, but she was socialized by the parents as well. The mother, an elementary school teacher, took her daily to her classroom; the father, a firefighter, and the son roughhoused with her. Her raisers socialized her according to strict rules for what is expected of a guide dog—habits of obedience, of relieving on schedule, sitting, lying still, and adapting to multiple environments—the home, the stores and offices of Weaverville, going camping and hiking with them.

When she was sixteen months old, Teela returned to the guide dog center to begin her formal training in guide work, which lasted for five additional months. There she learned to wear and pull smoothly on a harness; move from curb to curb, or point A to point B, as instructed; follow specific commands; find stairs and elevators; know her left from her right; stop at changes in elevation; clear both herself and her follower when moving through doorways and around obstacles like garbage cans, scaffolding, and parked cars; and dutifully show intelligent disobedience when needed—such as when her person might be in danger of stepping off the edge of a railway platform or into oncoming traffic.

When I arrived on the guide dog campus at the start of Teela's sixth month, I had to learn what she already knew. I began a highly disciplined four weeks in residence of doing as I was told—moving my arms and legs with prescribed gestures, using an appropriate tone of voice and select words so that Teela could recognize my wishes and lead me safely. We would walk the sidewalks of San Rafael with a trainer behind us, instructing me on where to turn and where I had erred: "Correct your dog." "Heel her." "Go back. You missed the curb." "She nailed it! Good for Teela!" I would sit in meetings with the often-heard command, "Control your dog!" as Teela nosed over to play with the dog next to her. At the dining table, for three meals a day, I sat with Teela at my feet, nose forward under the table communing with the other dogs—the big round table spaced, pinwheel fashion, with person, dog, person, dog—each dog attached to its user with its leash tucked under the person's left thigh so that a stirring of the dog could be felt. I kept alert for Teela's movements, knowing I might have to settle her at any moment. Sometimes outside while we were practicing our guide work, the trainers would walk by carrying a cat in their arms or extending a piece of food, such as a hot dog, trying to tempt and distract our dogs. I grasped Teela's leash extra tight, knowing I had a highly excitable, easily distracted dog and not wanting to fail the test of being able to control her.

For Teela was, from the start, a strong-willed dog, responsive to her environment, sensitive, easily aroused, interested in everything around her, eager to get places quickly and perhaps veer off to new ones. She was dutiful in doing as I asked—she knew her left from her right, stopped at curbs, and looked toward me for direction—but always I felt she conveyed a sense that, "if you don't watch out, I will just take you where I want to go."

In the training, each of us had to prove we could control our dog and handle the dog expertly so that we would be safe and the dogs would reliably work for us. Since Teela was so high-strung and energetic in the way she pulled me when guiding, I felt I had to do extra work each day to be sure she knew who was in command and in the hope of tiring her a bit before the formal instruction of the day began. I would go out with her every morning before breakfast in the semi-dark, walking the grounds of the guide dog campus, giving her commands, working with her so she would not pull me off course into bushes or grass beside the path as she enthusiastically marched us forward. Some of my most vivid memories from our time in guide dog school are of our walks those early mornings when no one else was around; the sprinklers were on watering the grass; the staff had not yet come in to work at their offices; the sun was rising, the sky glowing a rosy red color above the long arm of a freeway blurry in the distance. I would work with Teela, practicing our drills so she would obey me, respond quickly, not pull my left arm too hard, stop on command, sit beside me, lie down when told, get up, come to me when called. We would do our obedience exercises standing under a street lamp, the light flowing down on us. After completing them, I would reach down and pat Teela's head, then look up at the gentle glow of the sunrise and hope that our day would work out well.

Early on, in one of our instructional sessions, a trainer made a statement to the class that has stayed with me: "You want your dog to feel that the happiest place to be is by your side." For Teela's entire life with me, I have wanted, more than anything, for that to be so. Fortunately, I was given a temperamentally happy dog, so it has not been hard.

But especially in the beginning, I doubted my abilities. From the moment the door to my dorm room was opened and Teela and her leash were handed to me, the question immediately in my mind was, "Will she like me?" It seems strange to wonder if your dog will like you, given that dogs are so often said to give their owners unconditional love. Though my love for her would become unconditional, I always assumed that hers for me would be dependent on how I treated her. "Does she like me?" is a question I still have from time to time, though I know from the way she rests her head in my lap, her eager attentiveness, or her happy appreciation when I do something she likes, that by now I think she does. In the beginning, however, I had no such confidence. I was simply overwhelmed with the size of the dog, her forceful exuberance, her strength, and the task ahead of us—to move through the world with ease, to move safely, to have her within my control, to find our way together.

When I was given Teela, I was also given information about her puppy raisers. During our training and continuing well after we graduated and I brought her home, I kept thinking that Teela must be missing the family who raised her. It was a long time before I would feel that she was truly content to be with me, that this was now where she belonged.

When I first arrived at the school, we were taught by practicing with a harness wrapped around a towel, and by being led by a trainer rather than a dog. Three days later when Teela was given to me, she moved out of the kennels, where she had been living in a dog run, and into a dormitory room with me. She slept on the floor beside me on a fleece pad, ate when I fed her, walked the streets of San Rafael with me, sat with me in instructional sessions and at meals—almost all of the time, except for brief play periods, attached to me by a five-foot leather leash. The leash was usually doubled over—making the distance between us no more than two and-a-half feet—one end attached to her collar, the other held securely in my hand. This closeness, I felt, was a model for how we always ought to be.

I used to stand each day in the area outside the back door of the dormitory accompanying Teela, in the early morning dark, as she relieved herself at the far end of the leash, waiting for the deed to be done, and, in the very beginning, for one of the staff to come over and clean up after her. This was before they taught us how to do it—how to scoop for your dog without seeing by following the leash toward her and feeling the shape of her body. I would stand and wait and look over at Teela's golden, strawberry blond fur glowing in the semi-darkness, and I would think, "It must be magnificent to see her run." Since that time, I have seen Teela run many times, and it always is magnificent, even now when she is older and her strong front legs are doing most of the work so she is slightly more bent on the run, less fully stretched out while loping. Because my vision is limited, I see Teela incompletely as she runs and she easily merges away into the background of a field or beach, but I can see the sunlight glinting off her moving shape and I know that she is happy.

The month of my residence in guide dog school was a kind of cauldron. It melded Teela and me together and gave me rules to follow—instructions for how to handle my dog and myself from which I was not supposed to deviate. I have religiously followed those instructions over the years with but one major deviation: I play Frisbee with Teela. It is something I can do with her out in the open, and, because she is a dutiful retriever, she will always come back to me. She gets her exercise and we both enjoy it. The advice in our training was never to play ball or Frisbee with your dog because the dog may then chase those objects when tossed by other people, carrying you in tow. I have never had Teela chase someone else's Frisbee. We do not come across them very often, and hers is a floppy nylon Frisbee made for dogs, not the kind people usually throw to one another. We are generally careful, and so it has worked out for us. Still, I often feel illicit when playing Frisbee with Teela, as if we are in a guide dog no-man's land. When we are done and I put Teela's harness back on her, immediately all is safe again. But it always seems to me worth the risk, including the risk of my tossing the Frisbee accidentally over a wall or high in the branches of a tree as Teela circles and circles in search of it. The Frisbee may be lost, but Teela comes back, if only to ask me where to go to find it. When I first tossed a Frisbee to Teela and saw her run, I was so very proud that this beautiful, massive dog was mine.

When I brought Teela home from our training, I kept her attached to me with her leash for the first two weeks as we walked around our house. Often I hooked it around my belt loop. Where I went, she went. When I sat at my desk, she lay at my feet. When I was in the kitchen cooking or cutting bread, she was by my side. Only later was I willing to let her walk around our home without me—though, in fact, she continued to follow me closely and has dogged my steps ever since. Over time, she has become willing to lie in another room without me, but she has always been alert to where I am, as I am to her presence. When I stir, she stirs. When I move into another room, she gets up and follows me.

One of the first things she did upon coming home was to take our poodle's soft toys—a teddy bear and odd animals made for dogs—and chew them carefully, using her pointed side teeth to take out the stitches so she could get at the stuffing and eat it. I had to teach her not to take those toys, nor the small catnip figures of mice and fish that constantly move around the floor of our house when our cats play with them. Teela surprised me by being willing to avoid these toys. She has the dutifulness of a Lab. She tends to learn and train easily, except when it is something she really does not want to do, like coming when called rather than following her nose when out in a field. I tend to think that Teela's Golden Retriever part is her "party girl" self—the one that likes to play and run off, greet people excitedly, and generally have a good time—while her Labrador Retriever is her "dutiful" self—the dog who sticks by my side, obeys me, looks to me constantly for permission.

When Teela first came home with me, our house felt very small. She was a seventy-pound dog at mid-cabinet height. I was used to a twenty-pound poodle lower to the ground and to three cats down around my ankles. Our house is long and narrow with relatively small rooms that were immediately filled up with Teela's solid presence. The motion on the floors—the milling about that I was used to—suddenly became dense. In the present, I cannot imagine our house without Teela. It would feel empty. But back then, it was a new experience to have the company of such a large dog.

At first, our poodle, Esperanza, ignored her. She would run around Teela to greet me or walk under her. When I attempted to play with both dogs down in our basement, each dog would play only with me. Esperanza brought me her toy; Teela brought me hers. After several weeks of responding to them separately, I gave up and told them they would have to play with each other. They did that for a time, but never for long. Teela is deferential, and Esperanza will simply steal Teela's toy from her and run away with it. They have each kept their own space over the years, though they do often lie close to each other. My hope is that the fact of each other's presence makes them feel they have the comfort of canine company.

When I first came home with Teela, I had to learn how to navigate the back stairs of our house with her. These are narrow, steep, indoor stairs with not much room for the two of us. Because I am often afraid on stairs, I soon began practicing on these to develop my skills. Teela's puppy raisers—whom I met at our graduation—had told me they had taught her that she could sometimes go down stairs slowly. I was grateful for that and worked at slowing her down, though the slower pace on stairs has remained an incompletely accomplished task for us. Her raisers also said they sometimes deliberately stepped on Teela in their house so that she would be prepared for a blind person not seeing her and tripping over her. This gave me comfort when I stepped on her occasionally as she lay on the hallway floor near our kitchen. Her reflexes, from the start, have been so quick that she often jumps up and moves away just in time before I trip over her. Her tendency to do this hurts my feelings sometimes because she will spring to her feet when I get near her even when I know she is there and will not step on her. I often cannot tell if she thinks I will step on her or if she simply wants to show herself ready to go where I go next.

From the start when she and I went out, I was extremely happy because Teela has a brisk pace and smooth gait. When walking with her, I felt as if flying. I could look up at the sky. I felt free following my dog! No longer did I have to drag a cane along the sidewalk, making my right shoulder sore. No more exhaustion from long walks swinging the cane left to right. This dog—this new mobility device—could carry her own weight, take me places, make me proud. I felt I was a member of a special class—one of few people, perhaps only ten thousand in North America, who can be constantly accompanied by a guide dog. The analogy of a horse was very much in my mind, because Teela was big and wore leather, and I was attached to her, following her but as if riding her—her strength, her determination, pulling me forward, taking me places quickly. I saddled her up with the harness and we were off. I was akin to a cowboy—a cowgirl—not on the range, but suddenly adventurous, in the open air, natural, just having ridden in from the plains. I wasn't some sort of artificial person, closed in, making my way with small steps. I was a big person, a nature person, a woman who handled leather gear, a country girl in the city—someone out of the ordinary, here with my guide. I was no longer simply a blind woman walking alone—a handicapped woman who counted for less or needed help. I was a competent person not reduced to the trivialities of life. I got the big picture, I stood astride the world. It was now mine. I wasn't walking through it so much as sailing upon it.

As I set out with Teela each day, uplifted by her surge of energy, refreshed by the air hitting my face, we took many long walks, speeding by others, stopping at curbs. But soon the force of her pulling began to take a toll on my left arm and shoulder. I sought out a physical therapist, wanting to avoid further injury. The therapist followed behind Teela and me as we walked, watching us move. "You have a very long arm," she finally said when we stopped to discuss it— motioning to my left arm and the extension of it through the harness handle down to the harness, to Teela, and down along her legs to the ground. "It's a strain on your shoulder joint and your upper arm." She then taught me how to "brake" with my torso and pelvic muscles when I stopped at curbs with Teela, rather than absorbing the force of the stop with my arm. I developed a habit of dropping the harness handle at curbs, holding Teela only by her leash—so that there would be no pull at all on my left arm. I began using my pelvic muscles as we walked. This improved everything, and these are habits I practice to this day. They had taught us at guide dog school to keep hold of the harness handle at curbs, so Teela was, at first, surprised when I dropped it, but she became used to it.

I was grateful to the physical therapist for being so improvisational. In addition, I was pleased that Teela and I had attended the therapy sessions together. Everywhere I went now, we were a pair. Not only did I feel special because I was with my dog, but I felt others responded warmly to us because of her—because she seemed so beautiful and responsive, with that sensitive look in her eyes, the way she was always asking people to like her, engaging them with a wrinkle of her brow and an attentive, inviting stare. I don't see all this from their side, because I am looking down at the top of her head, but I know from her body movements, and from the occasional glimpse, that she is endearing—a dog others warm to. Before Teela, in public, I had felt unwanted and anonymous, like a person of no regard or little value; having Teela with me suddenly made me feel liked, as well as not alone, more safe and guided.

One day not long after I had developed the habit of letting go of her harness handle at curbs, I also let go of Teela's leash. I had been holding it loosely in my right hand when, all of a sudden, she bolted. We were on a corner on a hill in San Francisco and down she went. I couldn't see where she had gone—it was so quick and my eyesight so poor—but here I was, no harness, no leash, no dog. I followed immediately to where I thought she had gone and found a family mid-block unloading groceries from their car, the front door of their house wide open and a black cat in front of it. Teela had evidently chased the cat after seeing it from afar, and was now looking eye to eye with it as the cat puffed itself up and hissed at her. I reached for Teela's harness handle, stepping forward toward her. At that moment, she took off, running inside the house after the cat. I heard the sound of a cat yowling from deep within the dark interior, then the sound of a baby bawling loudly. I rushed up the front steps, through the doorway, and into the dark house—into what seemed the living room—caught a glimpse of my golden girl, grabbed her, and hauled her out—the cat opposite her still yowling, the baby crying.

When I stepped outside with my guide dog in tow, the parents were not pleased. A stranger and a dog had just entered their house and everyone was crying, and I had not asked permission. I could understand their distress but I felt, "At least I got my dog. What are you doing with a cat like that, and why is your baby bawling?" At times like these, I lapse into self-defense, and it is not entirely rational. I apologized. I said how sorry I was and left with my dog. Never again has that type of thing occurred for me. When I drop the harness handle at curbs, I now always hold Teela's leash tightly. I expect that a cat may appear at any moment, causing her to chase it. And there I will be again entering someone's house to their stern disapproval.

Sometimes when we are out, we come across a cat together. From the start, Teela has always nosed forward toward any cat she finds as if to examine it, pulling me with her. She never chases our cats in the house—in fact, she gives them wide berth—but these strange cats are a temptation more suggestive of wild prey. One day, early on, when I had let her off leash on a dead-end street, she ran after a cat, who stopped, turned toward her, puffed itself up, and reached out its claws toward her face, hissing menacingly. Teela then ran and got between my legs. That, too, was a lesson for me, that Teela would chase but not really eat the cat, or a rabbit, or duck, I suppose, that she felt was an appropriately sized prey for her. However, I knew that when I was in guide dog school, a returning student had told me that once when she let her previous guide dog loose in a park with a pond, the dog came back with a duck in her mouth. I have never wanted to find out whether Teela would do the same. Perhaps she would not eat the duck or cat, but she might try to retrieve it for me. And more than that, she was telling me, that day, that I was to take care of her in the face of threat.

When she was about three, Teela began to get white in her face, developing a Golden Retriever "mask" around her eyes and nose. She had been a solid strawberry blond before except for her white belly and white feet. Now, as her face began to lighten, people began saying to me on the street, "Oh, an old dog." Or, "I see she is getting old." I had just begun to move in the world with my young, exuberant guide, and I did not want to think she was getting older, or even that she was perceived as such. She wasn't old, wasn't weak, her best days behind her. She was only shortly ago a puppy. "Not old," I said repeatedly to people when they thought her whiteness was a sign of age. "She's three. She's four. It's the Golden mask. She started turning white at three. It's something that happens to Golden Retrievers." And they would nod their heads knowingly, unaware perhaps of the quickness of my defense of the age of my dog—as if it needed defense, as if I would be losing something if she was older—as if she would be less pure, less beautiful, less to be desired, as would I.

At present, Teela's entire face is white. She no longer has the Golden mask. She looks more natural to me now, as if the whiteness in her face, like the whiteness spread throughout her body—the lighter gold that she has become—is how she has always been—not a sign of her age but of her nature—a mixture of Golden and Lab, of white and yellow. But this betrays again my anxieties—about my girl growing older, and about the degree to which my sense of who I am is intertwined with her—and not only in her later years, but almost from the start. From when I first brought Teela home, when people said as we walked the streets, "What a beautiful dog!" I felt I was beautiful too, or I hoped so. "What if they give me an ugly dog for my next guide?" I have wondered. How will I manage? What will people say? How can I go through the world not looking good, not being as beautiful, tall, and proud as Teela, not inviting such a warm response as I have received when out with her?

It has not all been warm and glowing, of course. People have repeatedly asked, "Are you training that dog?" making me feel uncomfortable about myself—as if I am not who I feel I am, as if I am not blind or deserving of her, since my eyes move and I seem to get along well. Often, people in restaurants or stores, or when I am inquiring about staying in a lodging, have told me I cannot stay or be there with my dog. But these reactions, though difficult, have been easier for me to respond to than the inner struggles they provoke—the sense that I am perhaps not blind enough, or that Teela is perhaps not capable or young enough, that we are deficient in some way. "We"—that is the crux of it. What happens to Teela happens to me—the good and the potentially undermining, the doubt that can so easily creep in uninvited.

Teela, naturally, knows nothing of this. She is straightforward, all dog, simple though complex, happy as long as there are rewards in her day, such as our motion through the world, our many destinations, times for treats, for play or rest, for looking around, taking in the air and the smells. She can sit with me patiently on the sidewalk in front of our house for a long time as I wait for a cab. I will feel bored. Yet her ears are up, brow intent, eyes searching, nose twitching—probing the outside, the sights and sounds, attuned to everything—hearing and wondering about events that are beyond my ordinary human perception.

When I was in guide dog school, I asked two of the returning students, who were now on their third or fourth dog, what advice they had for me. The first, a man, said, "Don't let her get away with anything." I understood what he meant. If my dog missed a curb, I should correct her—go back to the curb, show it to her, tell her, "Careful," then redo the stop. She needed to know that you should never miss curbs. It had to be a deeply ingrained habit—a way of life for us both.

The second student I asked was a woman. She said, "If you have been walking for a while and haven't spoken to your dog, talk to your dog." That seemed to me such female advice—all about the relationship and giving support within it, not losing touch. It contrasted with the advice from the man, though both recommendations were good and I was grateful for them. At the time, I wondered what "for a while" meant in the woman's advice. Was it after a block, or after two? Why would we have to talk? What, in fact, would we talk about? I have heard her suggestion often in my mind as I have walked with Teela and as I speak with her—sometimes to give her a command, sometimes simply commenting on the day. She furrows her brow; she looks toward me attentively, her ears rise, turn forward; her body waits. She is considering what I have said. Am I talking to myself? I sometimes wonder. Is this truly necessary? Why not speak only when giving a command? But when Teela puts on her brakes, when she tries to eat candy that has fallen from bins in the grocery store, when she is tempted to smell the base of signposts where other dogs have left their scent, when she wants to race me to the pet shop when I wish to walk to the hardware store—yes, I need to correct her, tug her leash, tell her no, give her the command to move on. By now, though, it can't be simply commands.

Teela and I have a relationship. We have known each other for nine and-a-half years. Facing decisions, we consult with each other—as when Teela wants to go to the pet shop, and I want to go to the hardware store. We reach the corner where the decision is to be made. Do we turn left and proceed six blocks to the pet store, or go straight ahead a few blocks to the hardware store? Teela pulls left. I stop. I tell her "No. We can't always go to the pet store. I want to go to the hardware store. Teela, forward. Now." I give a small yank on her leash, leaning my body weight in the forward direction. She looks at me and turns her head sideways in the pet store direction. "I want to go there," she says. "Another time," I promise, "I will take you to the pet store."

She likes the pet store because it is full of good smells, with dog treat bins close to the ground; other dogs come in, and people make a fuss over her. However, generally in stores, she has always been impatient, thinking our purpose is to rush through them and get back out. When in the hardware store, she is bored because there is much standing around as I handle items of little meaning to her and as I wait for a sales clerk to help me find what I cannot see. When I finally reach the register, she noses up to the rear of the person in front of us, who turns around. "Sorry," I say, as if it is natural to be sniffed in the behind by a dog but also that it needs an apology. And we are off again to more interesting activities.

Teela has always preferred the bustling commercial streets as we walk rather than the quieter ones I like. When we do errands in our neighborhood, she has, from the start, slowed down on our return when I want to take the quiet route back. At the corners, she looks toward the commercial street a long block away, where, when she was a puppy, she was fascinated especially by the trolleys that run on tracks down the middle. She tells me with a tug and toss of her head that she wants to go there.

On our annual visit from our Guide Dogs representative, I asked about the dilemma. Which way should we go? "Don't let her take you her way," the trainer said. "She should go the way you want to go." This has helped me in having the confidence to make Teela return with me by the quieter residential street rather than by her route, which takes longer. Yet I often will let her take us her way—where she can watch the trolleys and get caught up in the general excitement, the air, the people coming and going. I will follow her wishes because I take pleasure in her enjoyment of her route, her more brisk pace, the sense of in-touchness with her it brings me. It is not me commanding my dog to my will. It is Teela and me sharing the experience. We walk for longer, and eventually I tell her we must come home. We must turn and again climb up the hill. But I know I have given her delight in her day, and it brings me delight. "We had a good walk," I can say to Hannah on our return. It was my walk, my destination, but also Teela's. We have developed a knack for this.

Sometimes when we are returning on a quieter street, I have tried to perk Teela up. "Forward," I say, "Party, party. Let's go to a party!" I have occasionally thought about tossing a piece of her food out in front of us so that she will whisk forward excitedly to get it. And then I can throw again and lift her spirit, make it soar, make her exuberant so she will carry me with her in that wonderful energetic way she has. But I have never done that. It would not be how you walk with a guide dog. The treat does not lie in the road ahead, in getting to a piece of food, but in the walk itself—in carrying your person along, taking in the air, feeling and seeing the sights and smells, invigorated—looking forward to the next excitement, the next good thing that will happen for you. It may be at the next corner, around the bend. It is definitely in carrying your person, doing the pulling, charging on, alert, up for things. It is in this shared pace, in life itself. I am happy I have had a high-strung dog, a dog with a love for life and a brisk pace.

Teela's pace is slower now when we return from doing our errands, and it is not because she is bored so much as because she is getting older. Yet still I am walking with my fast-paced dog. Any day now, I think, she will walk briskly again. And on some days, she does, nose up, high-spirited, happy. "Where are we going next? Can I take you to the playing field? Can I take you to the butcher? When we get home, can I visit the neighbor who plays with me and bounces a ball in her yard? When we get home, I can drink. I will go out in our yard and sniff and eat plants. I will go to my bed. We'll have dinner."

They say that dogs are present-oriented, so I am not sure that Teela thinks as far ahead as dinner when we come back from a walk. But I do think she looks forward to the next event, the next exciting thing. Only when we have gone out and come back too soon does she feel a lack in her upcoming destination—since she does not want to return from the excitement of being out. The house is interesting. It has food and toys, but it is no match for the wider world.

When Teela first came home with me, she was big and she filled up the house. When Teela first came home with me, she was a new experience. I walked the streets with her twice a day—long walks to be sure she got her exercise. Now I walk with her for shorter times, not wanting to tire her. And I often think back to those earlier days when she and I were young.

May 2013

THREE

✦✦✦✦✦

This Furry Companion

ONE DAY WHEN TEELA was nine years old and had strained her left rear leg, I left her at home to rest when I went to the supermarket to buy a birthday cake for Hannah. I walked to the store using my cane, moving it back and forth, grazing the sidewalk, noticing how alone I felt and how tired, almost from the start, because I would have to do all the work of getting from here to there myself. No one would call out, "What a beautiful dog." No one would stop me to ask how she was, if she was being trained, or how long I had had her, or to comment on her going white. People I passed on the street did not seem to give a second look to my cane or to me.

In the store, I was acutely aware of having the full use of both my hands as I took the cake from a shelf and put it in a shopping bag—where usually I would have only one hand free, the other juggling Teela's leash. Walking out of the store, heading for the bus stop, I carried the large cake in its bag in my right hand, my white cane extended in my left. I knew that if Teela were with me, I would be feeling insecure carrying a cake in this way—holding it in one hand, my other grasping the harness handle. Normally, my right hand should be free—available in case I needed suddenly to take up Teela's leash. Should a pedestrian threaten to bump into me, should I need to give Teela guidance around that person, should Teela attempt to go off course and stop to smell a fire hydrant or another dog's behind, I would need to use my right hand to give the leash a quick flick to "correct" her, to advise her to get back on course, to train her attention on our route ahead. Should someone try to distract my dog or to pet her, I need my right hand free to give Teela a cue not to respond. I need it to pat her head when we stop at a curb and I want to reward her for stopping, for not briskly walking on as we both so often want to do. "Good girl," I tell her and we proceed.

When I reached the bus stop, I finally cried. Here I was standing with a cake but no dog. The fog was thick, the wind whipping it, the noises of cars and other buses in the background. I cried in deep inner sobs that blended with the surrounding commotion. The bus took a long time to come. By then, I was done crying and got on, placing the cake carefully on the seat next to me—aware that, normally, I would be placing Teela carefully between my legs, sitting her down, reassuring her that our ride would be short. At my stop, as if she were there, I got off the bus quickly, dangling the cake in its bag behind me.

When I entered the house and went upstairs, there she was. Teela, who had no idea of the trials of my outing, simply greeted me happily, wiggling and wagging excitedly, her anxieties coming forth and now relieved. Perhaps, though, she did sense my tears as I looked down at her and stroked her head, tried to express to her what life had been like without her, and how I so wanted her leg to get better.

"I really do need a dog," I told myself after that. "I have taken good care of Teela so that she has had a long working life. When she retires, I don't want to go back to the cane. I will need a new guide."

Not so very long ago, I could not have imagined I would become dependent on a dog, that I would become a guide dog user for life, that once spoiled by that relationship—that sense of being not alone, of being guided safely, of having someone else to consult with at every turn—I could not have imagined how natural to me that sense would become. I could only imagine myself with Teela, talking with her, interacting as we walked along.

TEELA'S COLLAR TINKLES. The three tags attached to her metal slip-noose collar hit gently against her shiny necklace, making a tinkling sound. Each time she has received a new tag over the years, the sound of her collar has changed. Right now, the collar makes a high-pitched sound like that of a cat bell—a melodious, light, and lively jingle. Sometimes the sound has been more a clunk, more plastic or dull in feel. Her collar is hung with a rabies vaccine tag; a tag from Guide Dogs that gives her identification number (396V) and their phone number; and a third plastic tag that has my address and phone. The phone number on my tag is my land line because I made it when I first brought Teela home and I was not then using my cell phone as much. I keep intending to get a new tag made with my cell number on it, but I have put that off, not wanting to go to the extra effort, as well as feeling: "She is always beside me. It's not like she is going to run away. If she gets lost, I do too." I really should have a new tag made because, when Teela retires, she will be going on walks with other people. And, in truth, she does sometimes wander away from me, and I would want someone who finds her to be able to reach me. This little tag is such a big sign—of my reluctance to let Teela go, to imagine that she will not forever be by my side.

Teela's tinkling collar identifies her not only for others, but also for me. It lets me know where she is. I have had a hard time getting used to the changes in how the collar sounds each time I have added a new tag. It's as if the sound of my dog has changed—not something she is wearing, but who she is—her presence in the world. I am not quite used to the current high melodious jingle, though it has sounded this way for a year. The jingle of Teela's collar has saved me many times, because often I do not see her, but if I call her and then listen, or simply listen attentively for a while, I can find her. I think perhaps a blind person needs a tinkling collar. They did not instruct us about that in guide dog school, only told us how to thread the chain properly, but it is integral to my intimacy with Teela.

A further mark Teela has is a tattoo in her right ear that gives her guide dog identification number. She was tattooed with it shortly after birth. It is a light green color. I cannot see it, but I know it is there, marking her as a unique guide dog. I have never had the need to show anyone Teela's tattoo as proof that she is my guide. I do carry an ID card with a photo of Teela and me taken at guide dog school that gives her name, her ID number, and my name. People have never asked to see that either, but I sometimes will take it out in a restaurant when a manager makes a fuss to reassure them that this dog with a harness on and dutifully staring at me is indeed my guide and can accompany me. Occasionally I have taken my card out in airports, though they do not seem to need it.

Sometimes when I am traveling on an airplane, a person sitting near me has said to me that they want to take their pet dog on a plane and maybe they will get a little jacket for it and a doctor's note. They tell me about how attached they are to their dog. I cannot help but be sympathetic. Yet I also think, usually later, when the time has long past when I might say it—"But I have had to become blind to take this dog on the plane." That it really is not about the dog is something I will tend to overlook at the time, as does the other person. Rather than thinking, "Would you like to take your dog on the plane too?" the question should be, "Would you like to be blind? Would you like to have the source of the distress that causes me to need this dog?" But I do not say this. Instead, I continue the conversation about dogs—seeking to have this animal, this guide, this furry companion of mine connect me with the world, open up possibilities for conversations, rather than turn them into conflicts or close them down.

TEELA AND I HAVE ALWAYS PLAYED. I have taken her to grassy fields and beaches and dusty desert parking lots to chase her Frisbee and to run. I have dutifully picked up the wet, watermelon-red and bright green floppy disc, throwing it to her again and again until she pants with the exertion, the exuberance of it all, showing her happiness— breaking into a broad grin. She then lies at my feet on the grass, the Frisbee resting on the ground in front of her, held upright between her two front paws—those paws that are so like hands for her. Her strength is in her front legs. The back ones are more like props that hold her upright. But her front legs and broad shoulder muscles are her power. They pull her forward, grasp the seat of the car when she jumps up on it, the ground in front of her as she runs. They give her an extra surge of motion, propel us both through the world.

This past week, I packed Teela's Frisbee in my backpack the night before I was to be on campus to teach—placing it there along with my comments on the student papers I had graded, my iPad, and a pouch of Teela's garlicky flavored treats. I readied our bottle of water and her harness and leash so I would not forget them in the morning. I was looking forward to the next day—our time on the campus all the more precious because this was the last spring Teela would be guiding me to and from classes.

I am a fairly introverted person, and the public exposure I feel when on the campus can easily make me question myself: Do I belong here? Will people look down on me because my position is only part time? Will my hair stay flat; will I arrive to class on time; when I open my mouth to speak, will the words come out in a sensible way, and in a way that does not offend? Will people like me, respect me? Knowing I will have Teela with me is an antidote to my self-doubt. I think about how we will play and how we will walk across the bucolic campus, how Teela will look for squirrels and smell the air. I think of my posture—I want to keep my head held high. I will wear my dark glasses and my leather jacket. I will look like a proud blind woman with a proud golden dog.

In the morning after Hannah drives the three of us to campus, the first thing I do when we arrive is to take Teela to the Oval—the generous expanse of grass that marks the entryway to the university. There I let her off her leash. She springs forward excitedly, looks back toward me quickly for permission, then runs, pees, and bounds off, following her nose through the grass. I soon lose sight of her in bushes in the center of the Oval. I run toward the area, hoping not to trip, aware that I must be especially careful because Teela is not with me to guide me. I call her name, but she does not come. I begin to worry that she will wander toward the edge of the Oval where she might step into the surrounding street and get hit by a car, or that she will eat something bad for her and get sick. I call again, "Teela, come!" But I don't want to call too loudly and cause attention to myself. Why doesn't she come? Why do I so easily lose her? Then suddenly, I see a tail, some movement in the bushes. I run toward her. She turns and looks up at me: "You mean I wasn't supposed to be doing that?"

I motion to her with my arms. She comes to my side and we begin to walk the length of the Oval together. She stays with me for a while, then leaves and bounds off in a huge circle farther from me, lopes ahead, then comes back to check—as if the distance between us should never be too great. As I continue walking, looping back around, I see her golden shape occasionally, then lose track of it in the surrounding expanse of green. I concentrate on following toward the spot where I last could see her, never quite trusting that she will return, not wanting her too far out of my sight. Finally, she bounds toward me. I hear the tinkle of her collar as she approaches. I put her harness back on her and we set out for my office.

As we head across the campus, our joint decision making strikes me. Teela wants to follow a straight line, hugging the edge of a main classroom building on the Quad—a route that will take us down and up some shallow stairs usually invisible to me. I want to walk on a flat path farther out where there are no stairs. We follow my route this time. On the way back, we will take Teela's. Past the building, she weaves us across a wide, street-like path with bicycles zooming by us. Then she follows a sidewalk, then takes a few shortcuts among several intersecting, small, curving paths. These shortcuts are her idea on this route that is so very familiar, almost automatic for her, since she has been guiding me on it for many years. Approaching the student union building, she stops at the front stairs so I can gain a secure footing, then takes me to the door. Inside, she waits patiently with me as I order a sandwich. Does she know that part of it will be for her? I wonder. She stretches her nose up to the bag as we walk out.

We then head toward my office and have a choice about stairs again. I want to follow a flat route and urge Teela to the left. She tries to pull me to the right toward the edge of the student union building, where there will be two sets of stairs—one down, one up. Though her route will be shorter, we go my way. As we near a street, she speeds up and pulls to the right, wishing to veer off on a slanted path to take a detour to avoid a bus stop straight ahead. I let her, following quickly, knowing her fears.

In the office, we meet with students, then share my lunch. As soon as I take out the bag, Teela pops up from under the table, where she has been lying, and sits eagerly in front of me, perfectly poised, in rapt attention. I unwrap the sandwich, take a bite, then offer her a piece; take a bite, hand her some, giving her more of it than I think I should. But the day is special, we are alone, and it is nice to share.

I play Frisbee with Teela briefly on the grass near the office before we set off for class. I used to have a longer play session with her to tire her out so that she would rest comfortably under the seminar table for the next three hours. Now our Frisbee playing is not to tire her, but because it is something she and I have always done when on this campus, and it brings us great joy. I throw the floppy disc carefully, keeping it low to the ground. She chases it, retrieves it, her body quick to the toss, her nose in the air, showing her delight. She takes some water from my bottle, rests, and then we are off, headed back across the campus to the classroom. As we walk, I feel tearful as I notice that Teela breathes more heavily now than she used to on this route and her walk is slower, but she is happy to go, to guide. I feel we both know that we are at the end of a long haul. Or I know it. I wonder if she does. I think she is only doing what she likes and has always done before.

In the classroom, she settles quietly under the table while conversations swirl over her head. This quarter, there is another dog in class—an emotional service dog new to the student. Teela trains her by example, lying still. As I teach the class, I can feel Teela lying at my feet, relaxing, stretching out, reassuring me with her presence. Occasionally she starts to lick one of her forearms, where she has picked up pollen, causing it to itch from allergy. I tell her, "Stop licking," then I continue talking with the students. At the end of the class, Teela springs up as if called and rests her head in my lap. She is ready to go—as if a long dinner time is now over. Outside we stop at an area behind bushes that is covered with tree bark so she can relieve herself. Then she guides me down a flight of outdoor stairs that I have never quite been comfortable with. But now I seem to relax, using her as my moveable bannister. As we descend these stairs, I am aware that we are returning from one of our last classes together on the campus and tears again come to my eyes. I also feel a sense of pride in the world of our own we have made here.

We meet Hannah in her office and head back toward the car. There, Teela jumps up onto the back seat, where I give her one of the treats I have been carrying. She sits looking out, pleased to be in this familiar home, to feel protected from approaching buses. She always looks happy when sitting in the car looking out through the window. The happiness of my guide dog is so important to me. "You want your dog to feel that the happiest place to be is by your side," they told us in guide dog school. My side has expanded since that time. It's the length of a leash, and sometimes of a leash extended. It has four feet and a tail and a powerful nose and ears that bend back and perk up when Teela is guiding me. My side has much room for play, and sometimes my guide dog strays from it. It has lots of panic in it as I despair of ever finding her and as I worry that she may hurt herself. It has classrooms in it, and office hours, as well as walks along city streets and days in the desert and on airplanes and in back seats of cars.

My days on the university campus with Teela have always been special ones for us. These are days when our aloneness merges with the scenery and we keep each other company, make each other feel good in a circumstance not designed for that. But we take full advantage of the setting—the fields, the play. Teela leads me to good places in myself, rather than to feeling that I am not good enough. I am, in a way, an extension of Hannah's presence on this campus, because she has the full-time job. But with my guide dog, I am also myself, more myself than I would be without her. For she frees in me that desire to have a good time, a special time, an adventurous time, to share my silences, my aloneness. I will miss her when she is no longer with me. But I will also always have these memories of our times together navigating academic life, of those moments, small as well as large, none more important than those tiny decisions we make every time one path intersects with another. Do we do it my way, do we follow hers? Where are we going? What will happen there? Will there be good things ahead for us?

"Time for bed," I tell Teela each night. "Thank you for our day. Good guide, girl." I began that habit when she first came to me and I have not missed a night. She settles in her bed beside me, with a light moan if her back hurts. But always she settles, as close as can be on the floor. With my right hand, I can reach down and easily touch her, which I sometimes do later when I hear her squeak or mumble in her sleep—talking out loud in her way—little wines, little yips, telling me about her day, having her dream. She is running, I am sure; maybe there is a ball, a Frisbee, another dog, a threat. Her legs move, twitch a little. She is running in her sleep, going places only she knows—good places, exciting places—the secret life, the day of a guide dog, the frisky adventure. Even in her older age, she runs in place, her dreams belying the calm of her daily presence, in her dreams talking to me still—as I listen and wonder and think, "Where are you? Where do you want to go? Where is that place that has made you so happy?" Probably I was there with her, I think, but I don't know exactly where it was.

I have always kept Teela clean. The initial instructions in guide dog school were to groom your dog every day—to brush her with a stripping brush to pull out her undercoat hairs that can make her skin itch, then to wipe her down with a wet washcloth. I still have the dark red washcloth they gave us for our dogs during our training. It is faded and thin now and not the only washcloth I use for her. But it has special meaning. It has been with us for a long time. When I use it, I am back in our early days. I am handling a piece of material intended only for the two of us. Bending over Teela, my arms around her, I rub her with the wet washcloth early in the morning, up and down her back and around her belly, her legs, her haunches, under her tail and her bottom. When the wetness of the water hits her fur, there is a nice straw scent that I associate with Teela. It is her clean smell, her wet fur smell, and it is comforting for me. I have always felt myself lucky that my dog has this gentle smell.

I brush Teela's teeth twice a week and clean her ears once a week, as instructed in the school. She goes to a groomer every two months for her nails to be cut and her anal glands checked.

Every six months, she gets a bath—full works with conditioner. She comes home smelling more like the perfume of the groomer's shampoo than like herself, so I am eager for the scent to wear off. But she is—for all these methods–a very clean dog. This causes me some amount of worry because many of the places where we go— where she must lie or sit on the floor—are far dirtier then she is. In cabs, where at first I had her sit at my feet, I soon realized that this was the dirtiest place in the cab. I then changed my approach and instructed Teela to jump up on the back seat after I opened the door. Dutifully jumping in, her next step was to stand on the seat, lean her head over, and lick the face of the driver. I had to discourage that, though I am not sure how the cab drivers felt. But I would act as if, "Of course, she likes you—she is giving you a kiss." Or, "Oh no!" I would say, as if I was absolutely shocked, then, "Down, Teela, lie," as she settled beside me on the seat, her head laying in my lap, a resigned sigh perhaps emitted. "She's a very clean dog," I tell the driver, wanting to explain her presence on the seat, and off we go.

On buses, too, particularly in San Francisco, the dirty floor— sometimes muddy from rain and smelling of urine—has been a constant challenge to my sense of cleanliness. For Teela is so much an extension of me—my arms go around her and all that she has lain in; she drags it all into the house, into her beds, to my hands as I pet her, my face as I nestle it into her fur. We are one in that way, and my dog on dirty floors has been difficult to get used to. Often when we come home after a bus ride, I take out the red washcloth and give her a once over. We are back from the dirty, noisy world—and my dog is now clean! Then up the stairs into the kitchen. This is our home, our sanctuary, where the harness can come off, the dog can become slightly less obedient, more relaxed, more free. Though always there is that sense of bondedness, of lack of total freedom—or lack of as much freedom as a pet dog might have.

For Teela is a dog bred and trained to be responsive to her person, to control her more wayward canine urges—such as licking of her private parts in public, or romping when she is supposed to work. She is a dog who looks over her shoulder for permission for almost everything she does—"Can I lick the floor now? Do you want me to settle? Is this a long morning when you will be at your computer? Can I lie in the sun?" In part, Teela's looking to me for consent is because she is a deferential dog, a middle child; it is her nature. But in part, it is because she was trained to have her life specified, disciplined, organized around obedience—this is how we pee, on a leash, circling our person; this is when you play, when you can go greet a friend, when you can wander and eat plants. It is time for the Frisbee now, and not now. You do not smell another dog's ass on the street. You walk by. "Teela guide me. Take me there. Respond to me"—these are things so deeply in her training, her early and persistent socialization.

People sometimes think that guide dogs are magically able to read stop lights and know red from green and to take their person to the grocery store on command. But it is so much more complex— an interactive set of signals. I remember, at the school, thinking to myself, startlingly at first, "It is only a trained dog. She can be untrained." Over the years, I have worked to keep Teela's training, which has meant sometimes overcoming her natural exuberance, her wish to chase cats, to eat everything she finds, to follow her nose and her strong sense of smell. I have concentrated on keeping her good habits because I have wanted not to lose her—not to lose her ability to guide and aid me, not to lose that purpose she was bred for, her accompanying persistent presence. I have wanted not to lose her if she hurts a leg or breaks her training, or wanders away from me even for a moment in the house—if she strays too far from my moods, my ability to sense her moods, to reach down and touch her, to know what she needs.

SEVERAL YEARS AGO WHEN HANNAH, Teela, and I were in a pine forest in New Mexico on a winter hike, it began to snow. We had marked our way back with memories of fallen logs and paths through the woods that soon became covered with white. Teela was guiding me as we started out, traipsing up to the tops of hills seeking to find a good view. It was a light snow at first, a dusting—very pretty on trees and hillsides in the distance and very quickly fallen. On our return, we were lost. Everything looked the same. The sky had suddenly gone gray, the air was chilled, the ground unmarked by anything that would give us a sense of direction. Teela had no use as a guide dog for retracing our path, though I thought of letting her follow her instincts and that she would then magically lead us to safety, like a heroic dog in a movie. We tried that briefly, but she was no better than we were. Her job in this circumstance was to keep me level and upright and following Hannah—for the snow was covering rocks and small plants beneath it and invisible dips in the surface of the ground where I might stumble.

We wandered for nearly two hours in the white forest, Teela eager, beside me, head up, aware of the urgency of our trek—the seriousness of it. I remember thinking more about her safety than ours. What if we were out for a very long time and it got dark and colder—what about Teela's feet? She had no booties on to protect her from snow and ice. Perhaps I could give her my socks. She was big; it would be hard to carry her, I thought. I could take off my jacket. We could make a sling. How would I keep my dog warm and safe? But she showed no signs of frostbite or exposure. She simply did as told, her nose up, alert, smelling the air as if she knew where she might be going but wasn't quite sure. Eventually, Hannah, more practical than I, and more focused as a guide in the situation than my dog, began to follow the sun. Not exactly the sun—because it could not be seen through the dense gray snow sky—but she headed us toward an area of brighter light in the west. Over there, in the direction of that light, was the road on which we had parked our car and the way out of this forest. But how to get there—over some hills or around them? There were choices. Hannah made them for the three of us as we walked—taking into account that I was being guided by Teela so an easier route would be a level one, where I would not lose my footing and fall and Teela would not step on rocks or cactus hidden under the snow. We trekked in broad circles, wandering for a longer time than we might, a time that Hannah would like to forget. "Never again," she cautioned, would we go "off trail." Never again, I thought, would I expect that remembering a log across a path in the woods would lead me home. We finally came out far north of where we had left the car on the road, but on the road nonetheless—a cherry red SUV in the distance. I was elated, Hannah was relieved, and Teela was normal. She looked toward me for approval and seemed no worse for the wear.

Only the next day when Hannah, Teela, and I were far south near the Mexico border, walking on a dirt road near my favorite mountain, Big Hatchet, did I become aware that Teela had an injury. We were out in the open surrounded by cactus and brittle bush; the sun was getting lower, and it was time for Teela's dinner. As she jumped down from the car seat, Hannah noticed dried blood on her right front leg. I was shocked. I did not want to believe it. I poured some water on the area and found that she had a fairly deep cut. "What do we do?" Hannah asked. "She has dinner," I thought. I took out her food from the back of the car, filled her bowl, and placed it securely on the ground, lodged between my two feet so the bowl would not slip around as Teela lapped up every last bite. Then I began to want to cry. How could I have injured my dog? How could I have injured her and not known it?

The sun was setting, the sky becoming orange as we drove back toward the nearest town. As we approached the highway, I placed a call to our veterinarian back home. "Go to Walmart," she said. "Get some liquid bandage. Put her in the bathtub in your motel, wash the wound with soap, then apply the liquid bandage. I'd then get her to a vet in the morning for an antibiotic. She'll be fine."

The best Hannah and I could figure out was that Teela had probably cut herself on a sharp plant as she dutifully guided me through the snowy forest the day before. She had possibly kept her wound clean herself by licking it. She had not cried, not led me to the injury site. It was something I had not known to watch for.

That night, I was grateful for the bathtub, the soap, and the bandage as Teela lay beside me on the floor. As I reached down to pet her, I felt her softness and calm. In the morning, we took her to a local vet who got down on her knees and handed Teela an antibiotic pill wrapped in the middle of a small hot dog. We then went to the store and bought more hot dogs for Teela's pills. Since that time, I have always given Teela her medicines wrapped in treats. And since that time, I have often seen her in my mind glowing in the light of a southern New Mexico desert, her fur as gold as the setting sun—a small wound on her right leg, a big leap in her heart, an appetite for her dinner most of all. I have seen her in the bathtub as she placidly waited for Hannah and me to figure out how to clean the wound and how to apply the liquid bandage. I have seen her in my mind as I have felt her—always between my fingers—her fur soft, her steadfastness, her simple beauty and strength. The day we wandered in the snowy woods was not a high point for any of us, but it was a warning about how quickly weather can change, and a time of our togetherness as we trekked and took care of each other.

In that moment, and in others like it, I have had to realize how deeply Teela's life had become intertwined with mine. As she breathes, I do; when she is injured, I hurt. When she is happy, I glow with her joy. It's an odd bond, an unusual bond—no guide in life is different, no relationship less importantly tended than this one has been for me. Teela has been a guide to a new way in the world for me, much needed because of my loss of sight; a guide to getting older, and a guide to sharing my life. In the nine and-a-half years I have had her, she has been with me almost every place I have gone. When I have had to leave her behind, I have missed her. I have run after her when she has strayed, listened for her tinkling collar, played with her, worked with her, watched her sleep, traveled in cabs and in snowy forests with her, kept her clean and safe, and tried to share her dreams. Repeatedly, I have sought to interpret the small signals, the nonverbal cues, the ways she has tried, and sometimes failed to try, to let me know her needs. And she has been constantly reading me, picking up on my nonverbal cues as well as those deliberately learned commands. I step out into the hallway near my study and she is there, lying on the floor. She gets up quickly, "Where next?"

June–July 2013

FOUR

———— ✦✦✦✦✦ ————

Our Intimate Bond

OVER THE YEARS, Teela has been with me in countless restaurants, springing up from under the table if I drop a napkin or move a leg in any way that suggests I am getting up—eager always to let me know that she is ready for my next step. She has been with me in restrooms, in ladies' dressing rooms, doctor's offices, and mammogram exams. She visited my mother with me when my mother was dying. She has sat at my feet on airplane rides despite her wishes to "get off the bus" and always looking toward the front door. She has lain beside me in the bathroom in the morning when I am taking a shower, cleaning herself on the bath mat, then giving me a quick lick as I draw the curtain and step out.

She has stood with me on corners in busy downtown San Francisco as taxi cabs pass us by, seemingly unaware of the indignity I have felt. She has climbed countless staircases with me and slowed beside me on the way down as I worry about my footing. She has run with me often to catch a bus she does not at all want to board. She has stood with me as I take out a camera in a desert wildlife refuge and point it toward distant sandhill cranes. She has never tried to chase these cranes. I think they are too big for her, as are the snow geese. But occasionally, she has curiously eyed a sitting duck.

She has greeted every person I have asked her to greet with as much enthusiasm as if this person were her long-lost and most special friend. She has waited to take treats from my hand until I say to her, "Take it." It is a trick we have: ignore the treat, turn your face away from it, and eventually you will get it. She has lain in her bed patiently, then come to her dinner bowl when called and sat poised before it waiting until I give her the command, "Okay," it is now time to eat. She once ingested an eight-inch long piece of electrical cable, and once a full bar of Dove soap—each of which I later found in her stool and then swore to myself that I would never let her do that again—though, with her nose down as we walk and my limited sight, she has eaten many things I do not want to know about.

She has slowed her pace for me on hiking paths so that I would not trip and sped up for me on city streets when I have wanted to go quickly to do errands and to get my exercise. She has led me to the pet store many more times than I have thought we should go and with great exuberance and glee. She has eaten red valerian and other potent weeds that grow in cracks on sidewalks and sometimes in our back-yard. When she was a puppy, she ate all the strawberries on the bushes in her puppy raisers' garden. She has greeted her puppy raisers, when they came to visit, with her old wiggling joy, which made them happy to feel that she was "still the same dog." She has sat solemnly with two of her sisters when they and their people—my classmates from guide dog school—visited us—these noble dogs at first playing with each other, but then settling down, at home and at peace with their kind.

Over the years, Teela has strayed from me more times than I like to remember. She has not come when called and forced me into panic, and at other times, she has sprung to me when called—immediately, with no hesitation—confirming for me a sense of our bond. She has sat with me in concerts where I have put pieces of cotton in her ears so the music would not be too loud. She shook out the cotton, so after that, I stopped bringing her to concerts—where I sit close to the stage to try to see the performers, making the speakers too near for her sensitive ears.

She has sat beside the dentist's chair with me and watched it go up and down, unperturbed. She has stood with me in elevators where I dread being taken accidentally up to a top floor as I wonder which button to press. For in that small space, my fear of heights mixes with my inability to read the numbers on the buttons or the Braille markings. She has sat on the back seat of cars as I ride in front, jumping up on the seat or stair-stepping in, climbing to the floor first, then getting up on the seat—easier for her now in her older age. She has circled on back seats of cars countless times, making a nest, checking the surface out before she settles down. She has refused to come upstairs and stayed down in the basement of our house often because that is a place of pleasure for her, where she made a nest and ate and played when she first came home with me nine and-a-half years ago.

She has walked on beaches with me again and again, off harness, connected to me only by her leash, pulling me forward as I, too, follow her nose. She has barked only four or five times during the years I have had her—a deep, throaty, full bark, though not extremely loud. She has kept me from falling many times—I have only fallen twice since I have had her, and both times it was my fault when I was in a hurry and ignored her signals. Normally, I simply grasp the harness handle more tightly if, tripping over some unseen object, I begin to fall, or I reach down and steady myself by touching her broad back.

Over the years, Teela has stood by my side and refused to move at certain crucial times when I have wanted her to let me pass— as, for example, in our kitchen when one of the cats throws up her breakfast and I want to get to it to clean it quickly before another cat eats it, or when I want to rush to answer the phone. Teela is so accustomed to being next to me, to being steadfast and patient in that way, that my need to rush past her is not in her repertoire. Her place is by my side; it is where I am.

She has survived my bathing her in our bathtub, her golden hairs thick around the drain, survived my bathing her the first time when I did not rinse her completely, so that, for days after, she itched until I took her to the groomer for a proper bath. I have always felt remiss in not bathing her all the time myself—as if I should know and take care of her every inch. She has brought me her Frisbee, she has brought me her toys, she has littered the basement with pieces of sticks she has retrieved from the yard, she has found tennis balls on the street and has shown herself able to sequester two in her mouth at once.

Once when I forgot to pack her food while Hannah and I were traveling, as we sat in a restaurant for a late dinner, I ordered Teela a bowl of water and a chicken breast on toast, which I sliced and she dutifully ate from a plate on the floor beside the table. I have fed Teela many meals of white rice and cottage cheese to calm her system after her dietary indiscretions. I have regularly bought many large bags of dog food, transporting two of the fifteen-pound bags home at a time, lifting them carefully out of the car, amazed at how much food my dog will eat. I have washed the blankets that line her several dog beds many times, first putting my nose deeply into each to determine whether it smells bad enough to need cleaning. When I have put the laundered blankets back, I have felt pleased to provide this clean bed for my dog. It feels like a token of what she deserves—a nice place to come home to, a place of care and fresh scent after all her time out in the world, where the smells and noises are not as comforting.

When I first brought her home from guide dog school, the very next weekend I had a conference to attend in Asilomar, California, down on the coast. The morning after the conference, Hannah and I walked with Teela on a nearby beach. It was our first time on a beach with my new guide dog. "Do you think we will ever walk on a beach alone again?" Hannah asked me. I wanted to say yes, and I wanted to say no. I knew what she meant—what would happen to our togetherness, our aloneness? But this was the beginning of my life with my new dog and I wanted not to leave her behind. A few months ago, when Hannah, Teela, and I were again walking on a beach, Hannah turned to me. "I can't imagine walking here without her," she said.

I have been continually grateful that Hannah has opened her heart to Teela, welcoming her into her life. This has meant my often walking apart from Hannah—walking ahead of her on sidewalks as Teela speeds me past other people. It has meant that often when I walk with Hannah, I do not talk to her, because I must give Teela my attention. It has meant always having this third person around—this other being who needs care and responsiveness, who leaves golden hair everywhere, who must be settled comfortably in the back seat of the car before we can drive off. Yet Hannah reminds me: don't forget that it has also meant that people light up when they see us, and this includes Hannah too, and it has meant that I have someone else to watch out for me, so she worries less.

A week ago, after thirty-two years of being together, Hannah and I got married when same-sex marriage became legal in California and in federal law. "Teela will be with us, of course," Hannah said to me when we contacted City Hall to reserve the date—surprising me, again, with her inclusiveness. The day before the ceremony, we went to a flower stand and bought a bunch of white freesia, which I made into a corsage and attached, with gardening wire, to Teela's harness. She became our bridesmaid, our flower girl, smiling in all the pictures. Our ceremony was small—attended by a friend who read the vows, a witness, and the three of us. Teela's presence made the event seem natural and fitting to us. She has, over the years, made both of our lives richer, happier, and more complete.

Over the years, I have always protected my left arm, because this is the arm with which Teela guides me—the arm that extends to the harness handle. When I have had blood drawn, I have given them my right arm; when I must carry heavy packages, I use my right hand and arm, never wanting an injury to my left. I say to myself as I move things about, "Use your right arm, or you will not be able to walk with your dog."

When Teela and I are out walking people have often asked me her name, and I have guarded it as I do her. I tell them that when I say her name or even spell it, she perks up, waiting for me to give her a command. I will then often lean over and whisper her name in the person's ear, cautioning them not to say it in casual conversation within her hearing because I do not want her to become inured to her name. It is something reserved to get her attention. "We call her 'Big Dog' at home," I suggest to the person. "You can say that." "How long have you had her?" they continue. Or, once outside a motel in Florida, a woman who asked and received my answer quickly gave me the rejoinder, "But I know a blind woman and she lets us say her dog's name."

I have not got this licked by any means. It's something I have done one way, and that others may do in another way. But I have a high-strung, distractible dog—a simple girl who has become more complex—but who is always on the verge of finding something else more fun to do. I guard her obedience, her responsiveness to me— practicing our guide work with her, time and again, committed to the habits that link us so intimately. It has taken stopping at every curb, correcting, and doing the stop over when needed; it has taken a constant vigilance on my part to keep us from straying from what we are supposed to do, from who we are—me blind, she my guide, both of us watching out for our safety, guiding one another as we go.

Friends have sometimes commented that Teela is like two dogs: the obedient dog who seems calm and still—the guide dog, the Teela when she is working—and the wiggly, active, alert, high-strung dog who simply cannot get enough loving or petting—the Teela when she is "off harness" with them. She has been those two different dogs over all these years, never letting either one of them slide or change much in their constancy. But for me, she has always been one dog. I know what it takes for her to be obedient and I value that and take pride in her dutiful, working mentality and behaviors. At the same time, her playfulness, her alert, "party girl" Golden Retriever self is a joy to me. And we go back and forth between the two. Had she not that lighter side, her more carefree dog energy, she would not be as good for me, I think, brightening my mood, lifting me up, making each day a new adventure, offering me a new awareness of my surroundings. It's as if she says, "You owe it to me. It can't be all work. We have to have some fun." And then we do.

Sometimes when I have been playing Frisbee with Teela out in a field, when I have decided we are ready to be done—because she is tired, or we have someplace to go and more work to do—I will plan to take the Frisbee from her the next time she retrieves it. She can often sense that I am about to do this and she holds the Frisbee firmly, grasping it resolutely in her mouth, not wanting to let it go. I give a tug but I cannot get the Frisbee out. "Give," I say to her. She rolls her eyes up at me, holding tightly to her prize. "Give," I say again, yanking it gently because I do not want to tear the Frisbee by trying to take it forcibly from her teeth. I get down, squatting in front of her, face to face—nose to nose. "Time to go," I say. "No," she responds. "A while longer." "No," I say, "Give, now." I then pry open her mouth carefully, but prying nonetheless. She gradually releases the bright red disc. I take it and wave it at her, signaling that I will throw it one more time. I want to reward her for giving it to me and to indicate to her that every time she thinks I am going to take it does not mean I will. We enjoy a few more throws and finally I take the Frisbee, hiding my intent, and put it in my bag. Teela then goes off a few paces from me and squats and pees—as I have taught her to do after playing because the activity stimulates her system—and we are off. As we go, I think about how much her liveliness is a source of pleasure for me. When she plays, I play. When she works, so do I.

Once after we had played in a public park and had our discussion about the Frisbee at the end, a woman came over. "I was watching you," she said, "the way you talked with your dog." I was surprised and flattered—not used to being watched this closely but glad that someone had noticed.

Often on our way home from doing our errands, my fun-loving dog has stopped at the entrance to a playground two blocks from our house. There is a tennis court within it from which balls may stray and a grassy field and side areas where she and I have played over the years. She halts at the entrance to this interesting place in the midst of guiding me, looks in longingly, and refuses to go on. I cannot tug her forward, cannot command her; I cannot physically make her go. I must, instead, have a conversation with her. I reach down and pat the top of her head and say to her, "Yes, I understand, you want to go in. But we have to go home now. We'll play another time." I say this thoughtfully as I touch the furrow of her brow, and I must take my time so that she will feel listened to, heard, and understood—her wishes registered. We then proceed up the hill. My dog and I—we talk, we have developed our ways.

Over the years, Teela has always expected that the world will be kind to her. She has stood stock still on beaches many times, eyeing other dogs at a distance, as if trying to make out whether they are friendly. Once a big, black dog coming close on a beach barked and snapped at her and it took her totally by surprise. She is so deferential in her habits and behaviors that other dogs know it and she is safe. But I always watch out for her. "Friendly?" I ask as a person approaches with their dog, wishing to protect mine. In our walks on city streets, I have sometimes kicked toward barking dogs who seem to lunge at Teela. I have often wanted to stop and play with puppies on sidewalks as we pass them, but I have resisted the urge, wishing always to continue our discipline, our training—to keep Teela a good guide, to keep us both on course.

We have been safe over all these years. Before I got Teela, I was hit by a car I did not see coming while crossing a street. I was tossed up on the hood of the car, spun around, and thrown onto a sidewalk. Fortunately, I was not badly hurt, but it was a warning—"You are not traveling safely." After that, I started using a white cane, and soon I wanted to get a dog. It was an extended process of applying to guide dog school, passing an interview and repeated tests, proving I was capable. And then I was given Teela, my golden girl, and I started having adventures with her. Often, especially in the early years, I took her for granted even as she changed my life. I had to get used to being led along sidewalks, and to what people would say—"Are you training that dog?" "What a beautiful dog!" "What's wrong with your eyes?" "How long have you had her?" "What is her name? Why can't you tell me?" "Oh! How nice for you, dear," they would say. I had to get used to getting the dog food, and to having fur all over the house—fur I could not see, but I feared others would see it and think that I kept a dirty house. I had to get used to my black dress pants being covered with golden hair—"guide dog heather," they called it in the school. I had to get used to how to maneuver Teela when Hannah and I were walking together.

So many things have happened to Teela and me over the years, so many significant moments. The world has opened up for me and become a more alive place. My blindness recedes as a handicap and becomes a license to travel aided. Walking with Teela, I think about her needs often more than my own. And I think about how to make my experiences into joys—small joys—because I am with her, because that is what she likes to do.

It's been a long time that Teela and I have been sharing this road: the sidewalks, the country paths, the city and the desert, the beaches, the campus, the back seats of cars. It has been a long time and I never want to forget—not one moment of it, not the special-ness of having her, nor the select group to which she and I belong.

I have been a person who walks with a guide dog. I have had that privilege. I have been able not to walk alone, to share the adventure, to be led by another life. In this case, that life has been more exuberant than perhaps I am, and more attuned to the smells and excitement of the world, more cautious at times—a guide into my future, a guide away from my past and from the noxious stimulants, the harsh noises, the things I might not like about the city. In our comforting of each other, our watching out for each other's safety, in that, I have found respite and a home.

Teela has been my moveable bannister, my guide dog, my mass of fur, my delight, who comes suddenly to attention, my companion who tells me, "Don't go here, but there," who winds me around scaffolding and parked cars and lets me know when the construction ahead is too much—who takes me into new places and strange stores and buildings, and, because she is with me, I am not alone. She lends to me her stature, her exceptional presence as a dog going places where dogs are not usually allowed. She lends to me a sense that I am now more acceptable than I once was, that I am a person who other people will talk to, if only to ask my dog's name. She makes a place for me in the world and I make one for her. I cannot withdraw as much as I might, cannot feel sorry for myself as much. I must go out because Teela needs to, and I need never to go out unaccompanied. I have someone to talk to, with whom to share the road.

I will miss my dog—not simply any guide dog—when I get a new guide. I will miss my Teela, the girl whom I have learned on, my first guide, my golden girl, who has made me—a self-doubting, introspective woman—feel more outgoing and less peculiar. She has made me, a blind woman, value my sight and my blindness and forget who I am—and my troubles—as I seek to figure out how to speak to her, how to decide, with her, which route to take, what shall be our next turn? In navigating our life together, I lose my sense of the deep chasms of my own, and I am drawn into another world—a realm of concern with my well-being and safety, my pleasures and satisfactions, my making the place by my side be the happiest in the world.

As I eagerly wait now for a new guide dog, Hannah and I make the adjustments required for Teela's older age. We pull the car up close to curbs to make it easier for her to climb in. We don't overdo it, or we try not to overdo it, on beaches, and to lessen the number of times she gets in and out of the car and goes up and down stairs. We play with her more at home in silly ways: the other night, we danced with her in Hannah's study, singing to her—"Come on Teela, twist and shout"—urging her to be more carefree. We are trying to give her a sense that becoming a pet dog has its advantages. In recent months, we have left her home to rest sometimes when we have gone out to dinner—when I don't really need her to guide me and Hannah can be my sighted guide. But then I miss her under the table. Teela has the beginning of cataracts now and some arthritis. She guides me along streets, but for shorter periods, and I limit the strenuousness, wanting her still to enjoy her work. She is happy to guide and she loves her play. More and more, life will be full of play for her. But I think she will always have that sense of obedience, of responsiveness to me. She has been my guide for such a long time that our habits, our ways of relating to each other, are deeply ingrained. They are not something that just goes away, or that I would like to have go away. And I think neither would she. We will find ways to continue our intimate bond, our habits, our responsive togetherness.

Back when I was in guide dog school, at our graduation ceremony, one of the puppy raisers read a poem she had written expressing to her dog's new person what life soon would have in store for her. That poem, long with me still, had as its refrain the dog saying to her blind person, "Come, let me guide you." The words were simple, and only some of them remain with me, so, since that time, I have filled in my own: "As you walk on the sidewalks of life, come, let me guide you. As you face your daily struggles and things you need to do, come, let me guide you. As you wonder what you are doing here and if any of it matters, and as you stumble and nearly fall, come, let me guide you. I will be your eyes, your nose and ears. When you worry about whether you are any good and whether your abilities will fail, let me steady you; let me lift your spirits. Let me guide you through the world full of construction noises, and balls and Frisbees and cats, and places we wish we had never gone. Let me take you to grassy fields to play, but, most of all, let me guide you home again—to that place where we both wish to relax, to be as one, to have the walls surround us, to be washed and cleaned and comforted and fed. Come, as you wonder, as you worry, as you think of what I have gone through with you, come, let me guide you. Let me guide you to new places in yourself, to new adventures, to having me always by your side. And when I am gone, when I am no longer pulling the harness, I will be with you still. Come, let me guide you."

July 2013

Part II

———— ✦✦✦✦ ————

Searching for Sight

FIVE

✦✦✦✦✦✦

Framing My Pictures

I HAVE PICTURES IN MY BASEMENT that I am framing from trips that Hannah, Teela, and I have taken. As I work to align the first and then the second photos in their mats, putting my head down close to each, straining to see the edges of each large glossy print, I think about myself: Why am I doing this? Shouldn't I just give up? What am I, a blind woman, doing matting and framing photographs, even taking these pictures to begin with and trying to appreciate them? It is so hard to see them, to keep the edges straight. I should not be doing such vision-intensive work. It isn't right. I am ready to cry.

I so often want to give up when I feel frustrated by my lack of eyesight—when I feel that I am useless, or disabled, that I have nothing of value to offer, or that I am not doing what I should—what a blind woman or a person my age should be doing, or what someone else might be engaged in. My lack of sight complicates all my self-doubts and is an impediment. But against any negatives emerging from it, overwhelming them for me is a sense that I have been given a gift—a new lens through which I now see. My vision, though imperfect and full of blind spots, is revealing, opening new worlds for me, creating a distinct blind point of view. My challenge is to use my new perspective to see what otherwise I might not, to use it to contribute to the insights of others and to help me value myself rather than fueling my self-doubts.

Because I think often about my eyesight—what I do see, what I don't see, and how I should act taking my blindness into account—fundamental issues repeatedly arise for me concerning not only blindness but vision, the known and the unknown, the nature of disability, and the value of alternative ways of seeing. Because my vision is blurry when I look at objects from a distance and leaves things out, distorts, and darkens the world, I often must search closely for what, at first, does not seem to be there—for the invisible in any picture or in my life. Finding the invisible element becomes a reward in itself, like figuring out a puzzle or composing a pleasing portrait. As I try to identify what is not there, I am aware that I am creating pictures in my mind, grasping temporary moments of clarity before an image fades or a scene fragments again into pieces. I appreciate my surroundings more now than when I could take my vision for granted. I experience more joy in what I see. Sometimes I will take pictures with a camera to capture an image I want to cherish, or to see details later that I may miss at the time. Then I will frame some of these pictures.

One that I am currently framing, and that I especially like, is a photo of a general store in Portal, Arizona, where Hannah, Teela, and I went on a recent trip to the Southwest. Portal is a tiny town located near the borders of Mexico and New Mexico in the foothills of the Chiricahua Mountains. My photo of the Canyon Creek Store in Portal is a brown-toned picture, and I like the way it conveys the shadowy sense of the place. I took it one early morning just after sunrise when the light was gentle and golden. A glassed-in phone booth sits in front of the store on the right-hand side in my picture, next to a white ice machine. The storefront, made of dark wood, is somewhat junky looking, with signs for Budweiser beer, Coca-Cola, and local notices tacked up beside a front door that may be welcoming but is now closed. I am drawn to this photo of the Canyon Creek Store, but my fondness for it is odd because I had a terrible time when we stayed there—in a funky motel located just behind the store. Towering above the dark storefront in my picture is a large sign announcing, "Canyon Creek Store, Cafe and Lodge" in flowing, hippie-style lettering. Dangling below the sign, hanging from the building's eaves, are strings of white Christmas lights—pearly drops of glowing light sparkling against the dark wood background—a signature of Southwest desert places in winter.

On our trip this past winter, Hannah and I had planned to stay at the Canyon Creek Lodge for two nights, but we left after the first because wild, piglike javelinas wandering around threatened Teela, and the motel room was too rundown—the blankets thin, the rug a mangy gray, the dim lights flickering eerily while a rackety heater blew stiff gusts of hot dust through the room. I had planned for a more serene experience in this remote place—reached after driving up from a bare, desolate desert floor toward the towering granite peaks of the Chiricahua Mountains. Nestled in a wooded streamside canyon in the Chiricahua foothills, the Canyon Creek Store and adjacent motel felt seemingly nowhere. It was not a place I'd go back to, though I like removed places. But it was the idea of it more than the experience—of a retreat and of taking a refreshing shower, and of a store in which you could find anything you might need for a stay in the mountains, a stay away from the usual. I keep wishing to return as I look at my photo, despite my distressing experiences there. Odd, too, is the fact that as I stare at the picture, I can't make out the detail on the wooden storefront. I see only the square brown shape of the building with the hippie lettering of the large sign on top, the empty phone booth and ice machine to the right, and a stop sign on the left side—these features framing the store like weathered antique bookends. I took my photo from across the road, looking over at the store, wishing to capture the quietness of early morning, to register that I'd been there, to come away with something.

That what I have come away with is only partially visible to me now should not surprise me, but it does. I am always surprised when I cannot see something I think I should. When I first viewed my Canyon Creek photo after coming home, I was distressed that I could see none of the detail I knew was on the dark wooden storefront: the signs for Budweiser beer, soda, the local notices. I knew the small details were there, but I could not make them out beyond a blur. I am not sure if I even saw them initially when I took my picture. I was probably focusing on getting an image into the camera's frame, not losing parts of it, centering it. Last week when I began working with my pictures, I asked Hannah if she could see the details on the storefront in my photo. She said, of course, she could see them clearly. I carried the photo over to a window with bright afternoon light streaming through it, held it up, and there I finally saw the signs on the wall and the confusion of Americana that gave the place character. Then I carried my photo back to normal light and all the details disappeared, as they would on any wall where I might hang the picture. Hannah does not want to see it in the main part of our house because the photo reminds her of our very uncomfortable night, and of the javelinas charging at Teela. She says I can hang it in my study if I want to, which I know; anything we don't agree upon for the house can go in my room. But there are only so many walls. My study seems to me often a repository for all my memories, for all things that are simply mine, as well as a place ready for new work. Each picture I have surrounding me has its own history and emotional import. I think about their meanings even though I can no longer see the pictures well. They look to me like squares of color and light, a few bold shapes, the details blurred, lost to my eyesight but persisting in my mind as faint memories of important times.

My photo of the Canyon Creek Store clearly contains contradictions—between my fondness for the remote store in the Chiricahuas and my actual experiences there, between what I can and cannot see, between what I forget and what I remember. A second photo I am framing, related to that of the store, is of a javelina. Like my picture of the dark storefront, this photo, too, is hard for me to see. The javelina is gray and fades into a background of bushes that are green but look gray to me. Hannah took this photo for me because she could see the javelina better than I could and she wanted me to have a picture of it to take home.

Javelinas are small, gray, boarlike animals with compact bodies on short, thin legs. They roam the far Southwest deserts in groups, and the mothers can be aggressive when they feel their young are threatened. On our trip, I had wanted to see javelinas but I had so far only glimpsed a few of them briefly. When we arrived in Portal, as I got out of the car with Teela, stepping into the parking lot behind the motel, a string of eight to ten baby javelinas came picking their way toward us, surprising me. The mother followed quickly, eyeing Teela, circling the car to get near us. I was later told by the store owner that although usually skittish and likely to run off, these particular javelinas had been given handouts and were not afraid of people but were not happy with dogs. Like a coyote, they feared, a dog might eat them.

Teela had begun to pee and was squatting a few feet from me at the end of her leash when she first noticed the baby javelinas. She froze, then rose ever so slightly—keeping her bottom low to the ground, her back raised at an angle upward—a large Golden Retriever-yellow Labrador poised as if ready for takeoff. She had seen the baby javelinas, although I was not aware of it until Hannah called to me, "The javelinas are coming!" I glanced over quickly enough to see the backs of the tiny babies as they trotted away down a dirt path behind the motel. They were pink, I imagined, though they had to be gray. I was confusing them with pigs, which they are not; they are "peccaries"—wild grazers. But the combination of my inability to see well enough to locate where they were, combined with the deftness of their retreat, made me imagine what I could not see. When the mother javelina stepped toward Teela and me moments later, I was glad to have her close in my view. I did not take her seriously at first. I assumed that Teela was curious, too, and that, if she could, she would get close behind the scruffy mother and smell her rear. She would be unprepared if the javelina did not think her friendly.

Hannah called to me to get Teela away from the approaching mother and to put her quickly in the car so the javelina would not injure her. Javelinas have tusks, although I could not see them. Hannah could tell that the mother javelina was not happy and that she was set on discouraging Teela. I opened the back door of the car, told Teela to jump in, then got in the front seat quickly and sat there waiting, sad to have lost sight of the javelina up close, and feeling somewhat silly. Here I was, a big person with a large dog, sitting in a car—a huge piece of metal and engine—while a little tanklike animal with short, spindly legs simply looked at me and slowly approached. I was shocked that I had been so scared and wondered if I was as scared of the javelina as I was of ignoring a possible danger and of failing to protect my dog.

After the mother javelina sauntered off down the path behind the motel, I got out of the car and went with Teela into the motel office, located at the cash register inside the Canyon Creek Store. I wanted to check us in for the night and to ask the owner about the javelinas and what to do if one approached me again.

Behind the counter, a rough-shaven man wearing a flannel shirt and suspenders looked up at me sideways. "They don't see well," he said. "Try stepping aside. By the time the javelina sees you, you may be gone. The javelina will charge by right next to you. Then again, she might not."

I stood thinking—that scruffy gray mass could not see me well.

He continued, "It's not you. It's the dog. You have to watch out. They don't like dogs. They're like rats. People shouldn't feed them around here."

Then he told me that someone had recently killed a bear in the canyon. The implication, I felt, was that the area was dangerous and I was now forewarned.

That night when I took Teela out to relieve herself before we went to bed, Hannah came with me to watch for javelinas. The next morning when I took Teela out by myself in the dark before sunrise, I had her relieve herself right next to the car, with the back door open so she could jump in if a javelina charged. I had my cane ready—my long, white, blind person's cane—in case I needed to use it to ward off javelinas. But none appeared. When I went to throw away Teela's stool in a garbage can near some picnic tables beside the store, I bumped into several wooden statues of javelinas placed low to the ground near the tables. Fortunately, Hannah had warned me they were there the night before, but even so, when I got close to them in the dark of early morning, I wasn't sure and had a moment of panic in case there might be real javelinas mixed in among the statues.

I left Teela in the motel room after that, when I went out to take my photos. I did not want to be peering through my camera lens at a distant object and overlook a javelina coming toward us. Later in the morning, Hannah, Teela, and I took a walk together deeper into the canyon. When Hannah left me for a while to climb up a steeper trail toward the granite peaks, where I was afraid I might lose my footing, I walked with Teela down the main road, which wound through bushes and trees beside a deeply sunken creek. With my left hand, I grasped Teela's harness handle as I followed behind her, while in my right, I held my white cane in front of me, ready to swing it at any javelina heading for my dog. I was watching for javelinas, who were probably watching me, and listening for their sounds in the bushes. Secretly, I wished some javelinas would approach so I could get a better look at them. I did not want to miss them entirely simply because I was afraid for my dog.

I took out my camera occasionally as I walked, juggling it awkwardly in my hands along with my cane and Teela's leash. I kept listening for cars as well as javelinas, hoping Teela would stick close enough to the edge of the road to keep us out of danger, and feeling I must be a peculiar sight. I was carrying a cane *and* following a dog. Other people might not know that a blind person does not need both a dog and a cane to be guided, but I knew, so I felt I looked strange. Periodically, I sensed javelinas in the bushes, but I neither saw nor heard them. We saw a few deer. The sun was becoming higher, illuminating the bare white branches of the creekside Sycamore trees, lending a glowing light to our path.

When I checked us out of the motel a day early, I told the owner of my concerns about the javelinas—that I had not anticipated I would be constrained in my movements in exploring the canyon because I could not rely on my dog, for fear she would be charged by an angry mother javelina. The owner seemed content to have us go, as if his warnings from the night before had been heeded.

Had I better eyesight, I would still have wanted to leave the Canyon Creek Lodge after one night, for the shabbiness of the room unsettled me. But then I would not have had this particular adventure, nor been caught between my curiosity and protecting my guide dog, which, I was learning, ultimately leads to protecting myself. As we drove down out of the Chiricahua foothills, leaving behind a strikingly picturesque place with large granite peaks and majestic rock formations against a blue sky, I wished I had been able to stay longer—to see more javelinas, to have one come right up and eat out of my hand, to have Teela smell the behind of the scruffy little javelina mother, to add that to her repertoire of experiences. It was a fantasy, but it pulled at me, and I felt as if I had seen it.

Back down on the desert floor, we stopped to pick up lunch at a second unusual place, the Sky Gypsy Café, where I took a photo of Hannah that I like very much because I knew she was happy there. The sun was warm, but not too warm, and the outside deck on which Hannah stood made her feel protected and content. Behind her in my photo stand the massive Chiricahuas beyond a broad stretch of desert and low scrub. Although not visible in my picture and although we did not yet know it, we were standing in the middle of a glider pilot training station—a facility for specialist pilots from all over the world who came here to practice gliding, flying over the desert in delicate kite-winged aircraft. The Sky Gypsy complex had been recently built by a wealthy computer entrepreneur who had made his money on antivirus software. All around us were landing fields that seemed to merge in with the flat extending desert. Ahead, a group of molded fiberglass hangers for the gliders stood near a row of Airstream trailers made of shiny stainless steel that served as temporary living quarters for the pilots. Down the road, a formal restaurant was under construction, but here, the cafe we were in was intended as the community center. It occupied the ground floor of a red wooden building that also housed a small movie theater with an entry door next to the cafe counter, a computer center upstairs, art gallery-style abstract oil paintings on the walls, plush rugs, lavish restrooms with broad mirrors, and all of it well-appointed and brand new. Here we were in the midst of a harsh desert environment, in this empty space, this wide wash of a valley between two mountain ranges—the Chiricahuas on the west, the more arid Peloncillos to the east—in a land of rugged rock formations, hot sun, fast high-ways, and cracked asphalt roads.

How odd, I thought. How awful! I wanted the Sky Gypsy not to be here. But Hannah liked the sophistication of it, that it could be out of New York City with the abstract paintings, the cafe serving lattes, cheesecake, and calzones, rather than green chile cheeseburgers and Cokes—the usual, the local. The desert is full of things like that, I feel—anachronisms, oddities, things out of place—a Sky Gypsy Café, a woman with a white cane prepared to fight off javelinas, little statues of peccaries near garbage cans and picnic tables behind a ramshackle store seen without details as a brown square in a picture.

The day before, on our way to Portal, we had passed the turnoff to the Sky Gypsy but had not known what it was. I had started the day determined to explore a ghost town named Steins, reached by a little-used exit from the interstate, and lying just beside it, near the border of Arizona and New Mexico. When we got there, the ghost town was closed. Locked behind barbed wire were decaying wooden structures, old bottles, white plastic bags, discarded tires—all of this visible to me only as blurry shapes seen through the wire fencing, shimmering in the hazy desert sun. This ghost town was supposed to be open all the time, but the gate was hung with a heavy lock and chain. Hannah jangled the lock, with no success, then took my hand and led as she, Teela, and I walked toward the back of the dusty parking area, looking for an opening through the barbed wire. A long semi-truck was parked in the rear of the lot, its back door open enough so that Hannah could see inside. "It looks occupied," she said. "Someone's living there," and there seemed to be a cat. I heard a meow. Teela looked toward the sound intently. But no one came to greet us, except the wind, the interstate rumbling in the background, the dust rising in puffs with our every footstep, rocky slopes of pyramid-shaped hills darkening the vista ahead. We walked back to the entrance, where the crumbling structures and rubbish lay on the other side of the barbed wire, but we could not figure out how to undo the latch, or find another, secret way to enter.

"I'm willing to try some more," Hannah offered, knowing I had wanted to see this ghost town—though for reasons unclear. Perhaps I was in search of some nugget of wisdom or inspiration, or a hard-to-find treasure left behind only for me when the town was abandoned—a key to all I needed.

"No, let's keep going. We need to get some gas before Portal. I don't want to get stuck in the mountains with no gas," I told Hannah.

We got back on the interstate and headed to Road Forks, the name of the nondescript town at the intersection of I-10 with Route 80, the smaller road leading south toward Portal. Two gas stations stood at the Road Forks intersection. The first, the biggest, was closed, its abandoned pumps ringed with yellow safety tape that blew in the wind, making flapping noises I heard against the low background roar of the highway. The dull flaps of the tape cut through the air, as memorable as that vacant space, suggesting that something more substantial once stood here. The second station, across the road, was also closed. Gas prices had soared. I assumed that if a station could not sell enough gas to cover its costs at these high prices, it simply "went bust." Like the ghost town, the Road Forks intersection felt desolate to me, empty, abandoned, a windy basin of nothingness, of promise gone bad but for these two shells of stations and a trailer park ahead, and a restaurant. We pulled up to the restaurant first. Why was it called "The Shady Grove?" I wondered. No tree or shade seemed in sight. A big banner sign hung on its front, but it was not clear whether the restaurant was open or had also gone out of business.

Teela and I waited in the car while Hannah went inside to ask if they knew whether the store down in Rodeo near Portal still had working gas pumps, and if it would be open on a Sunday. She did not think we truly needed more gas, but I wanted to be sure we were safe. What if something calamitous happened to us and we needed to have lots of gas? In the restaurant, the woman told Hannah we should not count on gas being available in Rodeo.

"What did you see inside?" I asked Hannah when she returned to the car.

"Dark tables. I don't know if they were closed or just not open today. There was a store where they were selling knives. Maybe some cigarette lighters too."

Before we left Road Forks, we pulled over into a broad parking area that may once have served as a truck stop, or perhaps still did. I wanted to let Teela out of the car and to walk around myself taking in the scene. Teela was more interested in sniffing the dirt and the air than peeing, though she eventually did. As I stood with her in the rutted expanse of dirt, I looked over toward a cluster of spread-out mobile homes—tiny square dots in the emptiness, a mountain range faint in the distance behind them. Probably it was cheap to park a home out here, I thought, staring toward the view, my vision drawn to two small, almost invisible figures that seemed to be a father and a son taking out their dog, moving between trailers. I heard the sound of their voices and a bark, reminding me that people lived here—in the shadow of "out of business," near a ghost town guarded by a cat, in view of a blind woman, her patient guide dog, and her devoted partner, who had said she would go to the ends of the world for her but probably did not mean quite this.

We then drove on, retracing our route on the interstate for twelve miles to Lordsburg, where two gas stations were still operating. After filling the tank, we turned onto a smaller side road that eventually led to Route 80 heading south. Our drive took us past bare stretches of rocky desert, past the huge stone slabs of Granite Gap towering beside the road like tall, gray, windowless buildings. Finally we descended into a more hospitable plain, that sunny borderland valley with the Chiricahuas looming alongside it. Approaching the modest town of Rodeo, where we had hoped to find gas, Hannah slowed the car, pointing out to me a refurbished vintage pickup truck parked beside a sign, "Turn Here for the Sky Gypsy Café." The truck, painted colorfully, looked like something out of Hollywood or Florida. I strained to imagine what a restaurant might be doing here, and how could it possibly serve good food?

The store in Rodeo was closed, along with its gas pumps, so we drove on up into the mountains to Portal, where I met the javelinas, which have a significance in terms of my sight. But so, too, does the dusty closed ghost town of Steins, the out-of-business gas stations, the isolated trailers in Road Forks, the Sky Gypsy complex, the smell of the dust, the feel of the wind, the rocks everywhere, the sounds of the desert stillness—these are experiences, visions, moments in a vast pictorial, each telling me something about what I see, about how I can put it all together and what interests me; each revealing, as well, my fears, my needs for safety and self-protection as I wander with Teela in a world fading from my view.

I wish I had taken a picture of the emptiness, of everything I saw on those two days when we visited and then quickly left Portal, but pictures of dustbowls, of nothing there or nothing doing, pictures where only the smallest detail is meaningful and then hard to see, memories of rundown motels and skittish baby javelinas trotting off in a row behind a dark wood storefront, images of Teela beside me rising to see them—those pictures are difficult to take with a camera, and perhaps more easily imagined than captured through a visual, though maybe a true artist, a painter, or a good photographer could do them justice.

How can I describe things that are meaningful to me—the desert, those remote places I love to visit, traveling with Hannah and with Teela, seeing somewhat but seeing only part of what is there? How can I find a perspective that will be useful, insights that will last? I try with my words and sometimes with pictures. I have pictures in my basement that I am framing from trips that Hannah, Teela, and I have taken. They will soon be ready to go up on our walls. One is of a javelina, one is of the Canyon Creek Store, and one of Hannah smiling outside on the deck of the Sky Gypsy, sun on her face, the Chiricahuas in the background. These pictures represent the significance of things I see and of feelings I wish to keep. They represent my desires to go places other people do not go, to share other worlds, to wander half blind, yet still seeking to see, to experience the far away and bring it close. In my pictures, I am guided by a loving partner and an eager dog as I savor things left behind, the isolated, the individual, the singular that stands out that I treasure because it is different—making me feel that I, too, am treasured, singular, and alive. I wrestle my pictures from the invisibility around me, and they are all the more meaningful to me because of that. I am speaking, of course, not only of the visual images I hang on my walls but of those I keep in my mind, framed through the details of the memories that surround them.

October 2008

SIX

✦ ✦✦✦ ✦

In Search of a Camera

I HAVE BEEN SEARCHING for a new camera that will enable me to see my pictures right after I have taken them, to discard the mistakes and improve my technique—my ability not only to take pictures but to see the world around me. My quest for this camera has been full of uncertainties about what I can see, who I am, and what will make me happy.

I currently have a 35 millimeter film camera, a single-lens reflex model with a telephoto lens that I have had since almost before I began to lose my sight, since that time eleven years ago when I was not yet fully aware of the impending loss. I remember the first time I used my film camera. Hannah and I were on a visit to the desert bird refuge in New Mexico that I so like. The telephoto lens brought the birds up wonderfully close, defining them sharply. Flocks of white snow geese with black-tipped wings were suddenly filling my field of view. I was amazed and happy. Since then, I have used my film camera on each of our trips to the desert, taking pictures of landscapes, birds, luminarias at night, seeking ever new vistas and possibilities, walking out in the very early morning even in the cold of winter to capture the glowing orange and red colors of a sunrise.

Last year, I brought with me a small point-and-shoot digital camera to try out the new technology. By accident, I set the options slightly off, so my pictures came out grainy. But I enjoyed seeing them right away on the bright screen on the camera's back. Throughout our trip, I kept studying my pictures and the camera instruction manual, using my ten-power pocket magnifier, holding it up to the booklet and the camera to see the settings and to read the instructions. On returning home, I enlarged my photos on my computer screen and examined them further, trying to improve my technique, enjoying each image no matter how irregular. I liked learning the vocabulary of digital photography and soon wanted to take the next step of buying a more advanced digital camera—a single-lens reflex model with a larger screen and an improved optical viewfinder that would enable me both to see more clearly and to take better pictures.

Conflicting with my desire, however, was my sense that it would be a waste to spend so much money on an advanced camera when I have impaired eyesight, and because I usually take pictures seriously only once a year on our trips to the desert. There, I use my camera to frame what I might see—singling out parts of the landscape, enlarging the image, drawing it in with the telephoto lens; then I snap a picture, wishing to bring home pieces of those vast, haunting desert scenes that mean so much to me—the broad mountains and mesas, the singular yucca and cactus against the wide blue sky. The camera with a telephoto lens helps clarify these images for me, enabling me to see them better than I can with my naked eye, to enjoy what otherwise would be largely a fuzzy scene with shapes blending into one another.

In my search for a new camera through which I hope to savor such images, I have been considering the size and quality of the lens, the number of megapixels I might need, noise, dynamic range, and the different models, wanting to make my purchase appropriately. I have focused on the qualities of the imaging device, overlooking, usually, the aspects of my eyesight that lead me to want to see in a more precise way. I have tended to treat myself as if I am sighted in my search, rather than treating myself as if I am blind. I have had a hard time emotionally reconciling the two seemingly contradictory conditions. It has been a challenge both to accept my desire to enjoy the sight I still have and, at the same time, to take my blindness into account—to work around it, to "see" it—this invisible presence that never really leaves me, even when I think it does, that seems, at times, a stumbling block but is always more than that. It is a deep mark on my identity, my sense of self, altering my inner life in its own peculiar ways, shaping my intimacies with those around me as well as with myself, and causing me often to question my identity. Am I sighted or blind? How do people see me? How can I best see myself?

Several months ago, wanting a new aid for my sight, I began to visit camera stores. The first was a small shop where, when I walked in with Teela and asked to be shown cameras, I felt immediately out of place. Here I was in a setting intended for the sighted, accompanied by a guide dog signifying I was blind. I told Teela to lie on the floor at my feet. The saleswoman handed me a camera to try. I lifted it to my eye, but saw only black. I could not find the viewfinder—the small indented square of glass on the camera's back through which I would have to see. I moved my eye to various parts of the camera surface, searching for the finder. Finally, I felt around with my finger, located the small square, put my eye to my finger, and saw light. It illumined storefronts across the street. The storefronts looked tiny and dark to me and appeared to be in black and white. I asked the saleswoman if this camera showed color, thinking it might be defective. She held it up to her eye and said she saw color, that the camera was fine. I took it back and pointed it at Teela close at my feet and snapped a picture of her. On playback, there she was—bright golden, filling the glossy, square display, harness on, her alert face looking up at me. I was so happy to see her—my dog, colorful, large, and clear. I took a few more photos of her, then tried again to see the stores across the street, but their images remained dull; the letters of signs above the store windows looked blurred and wavy, unreadable to me. I handed the camera back to the sales clerk and walked out of the shop, feeling disappointed that I had not been able to see through it better.

A few days later, I visited a larger professional camera store housed in a huge warehouse building. Again feeling self-conscious about arriving with a guide dog, I walked up to a long glass counter and asked a sales clerk if I could handle some cameras. I told him I was interested in a single-lens reflex model and that I needed a good telephoto lens because I could not see well. He lifted several cameras from the glass case behind him, attached their lenses, and handed one to me. I had trouble seeing through the camera in what, for me, was the dark interior of the store, so I asked him if I could step outside. The salesman then followed me as I followed Teela toward the sunlight beyond the store's front door. Standing out in the parking lot, he handed me one of the two cameras he had been carrying for me. Holding it up to my right eye, I struggled to find the viewfinder, apologized to the salesman for my difficulty, put my finger to where I thought the finder should be, put my eye to my finger, and finally peered through the lens. There I saw a large building that looked tiny and colorless, with blurred windows and doors. I wondered if my eye was blurring the image or if the camera was at fault. I told the salesman, who instructed me to use the diopter adjustment on the camera. But I could not find it. The camera back looked totally black to me, and although I could feel bumps and dials, I did not want to press in the wrong place. I asked if he could put my finger on the diopter adjuster. He did. I moved it, but I still could not get an image to become clear.

I pressed the shutter button, hoping that would help, but the camera focused so quickly, while my eye moved so slowly, that I could not keep up. The picture was gone before I could see it. I began to feel dismayed. I was used to a film camera that focused more gradually, enabling me to see my images becoming clear before the shutter clicked. I had always liked the experience of witnessing a picture emerging into sharpness from an initial blurriness—as if my eyesight itself was suddenly repairing. But now that pleasure seemed beyond me.

"Maybe if you take the camera inside," the salesman offered. "There's a large sign for the store on the wall. You can focus on it to set the diopter adjustment."

He led the way as Teela followed him and I followed her. Inside, I pointed the camera toward the store's sign, but I still had trouble seeing. I handed the camera to the salesman and asked if he could adjust the diopter setting to what looked good for his eye, and maybe that would help my eye too. Odd as it may sound, having his setting seemed to me better than having no diopter adjustment at all. He moved the adjuster dial, handed the camera back to me, and we stepped outside once more.

In the parking lot, I directed the camera again toward the far building. I pressed the shutter button. The camera clicked off four shots in quick succession before I could stop it. I looked toward the salesman, wishing not to have to ask his help—not to have to seem to need extra because I could not see well—yet wishing so much that this camera model would work out for me. "It's the multishot," he said and began instructing me on how to turn it off. "Look for the multisquared icon on the back," he said. I could not see the small icon and wondered why he thought I should be able to. I handed the camera back to him to fix it, then took it once more. I was now all too self-conscious about the time I was taking trying out cameras and acutely aware of the three of us standing there outside the store's front door—Teela, my beautiful golden guide, wagging her tail at each new customer who came or went, the patient salesman standing at a respectful distance from us, spare camera in hand, me struggling, eye to finder, peering into the unknown, waiting for an image to become clear.

After several more tries and my snapping pictures of car license plates and a chain-linked fence, we returned inside. At the counter, I stood waiting for another salesman to take over while the first salesmen went to attend to a prior commitment. Teela lay on a rug at my feet, interested in the activities of people bustling around her. A customer soon came up to ask if he could take her picture to test out a camera. I instructed her to stay still. He happily snapped her photo. When done, he asked if he could pet her. Although I told him no, that she was working, I felt reassured by his friendliness, and I felt as if his recognition of her was also a recognition of me and perhaps an acceptance, which helped to counter my feelings of awkwardness about being a blind woman with a guide dog in a camera store. After that, I took several photos of Teela myself, glad to see her golden shape filling the glossy camera screen.

A second salesman then arrived to show me additional telephoto lenses, attaching one to a camera. I looked through the long lens toward the front door but could not see color. A third salesman took over to write down information for me about the models and their pricing. I was then more worried that the sales staff would think I planned to buy a camera online, rather than in the store, than I was worried about appearing peculiar because I had a guide dog yet was trying out cameras. As I left the professional camera store following Teela toward the street, I felt confused about my choices—one of the camera models I had liked had a good zoom, but it was stiff; another shot the images too quickly. I couldn't see the pictures becoming clear in either camera. I could not see colors well. I couldn't set the diopter adjustment or make out the icons. I wasn't sure what to do. At the same time, I felt proud of myself for trying, for getting to the professional camera store at a distance from my home, for overcoming my self-consciousness about my contradictory identity—my being blind enough to need a guide dog, yet sighted enough to want to take pictures. I had to ask for help. I had to deal with not seeing as clearly as I wished. I was still unsure about which camera and lenses would be best for me, but I now had better knowledge.

A few weeks later, I visited yet another camera store, located near the university. This was a well-to-do photography store with long-time, knowledgeable staff. I was now seeking further advice to help finalize my decision. Unfortunately, as Teela and I approached the counter, the salesman who came up to greet us did not have the expertise I needed, or it was hidden beneath a diffident and condescending attitude. He sized me up as requiring a more minimal camera than I wanted and handed me two models, neither of which I could see through, because their viewfinders were too small and dark. Begrudgingly, he took me to the Nikons. He mumbled a bit about this being one of their better camera lines, as if implying that it was not intended for a person like me. I asked for a specific model and lens that I wanted to try, carried the camera to the broad front window of the store, and looked out at yet another street scene—at stores across the way, cars on the road, hubcaps, license plates, and a tall tree farther away—pulling it all into view with the telephoto. There was good light coming through the window, bright but not too glaring, enabling me to see better than I had expected. I now knew how to find the optical viewfinder with my finger first, then put my eye to it. I was getting good at trying out cameras. This Nikon model, a D90, felt comfortable in my hands, the solid clunk of the shutter was reassuring. The stubby telephoto focused not as quickly as the previous lenses had. I could almost see the image becoming sharp. I thought that if I bought this camera, with both a portrait and a telephoto lens, I would be okay.

I also was planning to recommend a camera model to my sister, who wanted one for her upcoming birthday. On entering the store, I had mentioned to the salesman that I was looking for a camera for my sister as well as myself, as if that would make it seem more likely that I would buy one. I now felt I could safely recommend this model to my sister, with the exact lens to be determined later, though she would probably not need a telephoto, since she did not have impaired eyesight.

Teela was lying at my feet while I handled the camera. She was chewing on something. I reached down, put my hand into her mouth, and pulled out a black metal wire twist tie that she had found on the floor. I took several pictures of her, returned the camera to the salesman, and left the shop feeling more settled than I had in a long time concerning my possibilities for taking pictures.

In the next week, I stopped into an electronics chain store and tried out some less expensive cameras. One had an ultrazoom lens through which I focused on Teela and then left her image on yet another memory card. When all else failed, I could always take pictures of my guide dog. I liked seeing her golden shape on the bright screen. It was hard for me to comprehend that with such a colorful picture displayed, the actual image inside this cheaper camera would not be very good. For better quality, I would need to spend more money. That was difficult for me to justify—both because I felt I took pictures too infrequently and because I expected that my eyesight would be getting worse, so that a camera I bought and could see through now might not be useful later. It seemed exorbitant to spend so much on an advanced camera. These were for people with good eyesight who could see the icons and manipulate the fine points of their vision to take impressive pictures. Still, I wanted to do just that. I wanted not to lose my abilities. I wanted to take good photos and to extend my sight.

I have not, thus far, bought a new digital single-lens reflex camera, although I now know which model I would choose and which two lenses. I have priced out the components, but buying the camera seems too big a step. I did use my knowledge to make a recommendation to my sister. She feels the recommendation is gift enough, but I also sent her a check to contribute, in a physical way, to her purchase of the lens. When she takes her pictures, I want her to feel I am with her, that I am part of something that makes her happy. Both of us have a fondness for taking photographs that I think we inherited from our father. He painted, drew, and took photos most of the time when he was not working—activities that made him happy.

Thus even though I cannot see well, I still find pleasure in ways I learned as a child, as does my sister, though she takes different kinds of pictures than I do. She likes photographing people—her family and people in other countries when she travels—while I like to take landscapes, buildings, sunrises, big things that don't move and that are not as overloaded with interpersonal emotions.

When and if I eventually purchase a new camera, I plan to get exactly what I recommended for my sister: the same camera, the same high-quality portrait lens, the same filter on the lens, and I will add a telephoto with longer reach to aid my eyesight. I will also get an extra battery and a case. My sister likes carrying her camera around without a case, just putting it in her purse. But I am more cautious, more worried about damage and running out of power, more worried about calamities. I think it is sometimes easier to get a gift for someone else than for oneself, easier to be generous, to honor an underlying desire.

In two weeks, when Hannah, Teela, and I travel in the desert visiting some of my favorite places, I plan to take my film camera, and I hope it will give me good pictures. I am going to underexpose some of the broad landscapes so they do not become washed out. I hope I have gained some expertise from studying digital technology that will improve my film photo taking. I wish I had the nerve to purchase a new camera in time for our trip, but it is just too daunting a step, too full of my self-questioning. Yet it highlights the dream— my wish to see better, to create lasting, vivid, clear images.

When we are in the desert and I get up early that first morning to see a sunrise, will I wish then that I had purchased a new camera? Will I feel content waiting until I return home to see my images become developed? Or will I be on the verge of tears, feeling I am missing out? I hope to find new opportunities, new visions, new ways of seeing amidst my blindness, to enjoy the vision I now have, even though it is limited. I am going to use my small point-and-shoot camera for indoor photos, my big camera for outdoors. I will focus on what I can see. It feels less lonely to have a camera with me. It is a companion. Like a guide dog, it's both an aid for my sight and a reminder of my blindness. It causes me to stop and look around, to focus closely when needed, to be aware of my surroundings as I take my steps, many of them not clear. But the important thing is that I am taking these steps, exploring the possibilities, not letting my blindness, my awkwardness, my sometimes sight diminish me. It is hard to go against the grain, to want to see when blind. And yet I do.

November 2008

SEVEN

‣ ◆◆◆◆ ‣

On Not Seeing the Ground

I AM IN THE MOGOLLON MOUNTAINS in the village of Pinos Altos, once a mining town, now a community of homes, a stopping-off place for visitors to the Gila National Forest. It is December and cold outside at 6:10 a.m. as I step out without Teela, but I hardly feel the cold. I have just taken a shower and bundled up. I am carrying my camera, ready to watch the sunrise. I am also carrying my white blind person's cane. I tap the ground with it as I walk. I want to find the right spot from which I can see the color changing in the sky when the first few rays of light appear, creating that gorgeous light show before sunrise that I look for every winter when we visit the desert.

Two years ago, after debating whether to do it, I finally bought a digital single-lens reflex camera with a strong telephoto lens. I had hesitated to buy it because I questioned why I, a blind woman, should have an advanced camera. But I soon took the step, wanting to stretch the limits of my sight, to take pictures that would enable me to enjoy what I still could see, and to see it better. With the telephoto lens, I magnify my surroundings. I enlarge my photos on my computer screen when I get home, where I see more than I did when I took each photograph. I appreciate and remember more and take comfort from my vision. I find excitement in the process of creating pictures, of bringing a scene out of invisibility into clarity.

As I stood in the darkness this morning in Pinos Altos, I could look through my camera lens at the pinpoint of light beginning to glow in the distant sky and at the clouds changing color from deep pink to orange that seemed so nearby—because I was high up in the hills and among them. I could see these clouds: huge, looming, colorful. I could see the dark blue dawn sky becoming tinged with deep red stripes. And yet, I could not see the ground. The ground where I was standing and attempting to walk was rough with stones in places where I might fall if I was not careful. It was a good dirt road for cars and for people walking in the daylight, and for people who could see. But this ground felt treacherous to me in the very early morning, in the darkness from the night but for the gleam in the not too distant sky.

My path on this dirt road would take me first slightly up a hill, and then downhill, where the road would curve a bit, then climb again. On the shoulders were ruts, barbed wire fences marking yards and people's property; there were bushes and low roadside vegetation. In my blindness, I could not see the rocks, the way the road curved, the plants, the barbed wire, the places where my toe might catch and I might fall. I took each step carefully, and I feared getting lost, veering off as I might were I driving a car in the night and the road was pitch black and I could not see.

Why do I do this year after year? I go out alone in the dark, simply with my cane—not even my dog, for I do not want her to get cold standing around while I take out my camera, point it toward that bright glow in the sky, zoom in with my telephoto, look at the back LCD display, and adjust the light—seeking to find that exact spot of focus and distance that will make the colors more alive in the picture than in what I can see with my naked eye. That will make this morning memorable, this walk during which I hardly walk, take only careful, small steps, worried that I cannot follow a straight line—which I cannot, without guidance—and the line here on the road is not straight. It's a winding country dirt road with ruts and rocks and vegetation by the sides, and a wrong turn will take me into someone's driveway, then near their house, and their dogs will bark.

Why do I not give up, stop trying to take in the world like a sighted person, stop trying to manipulate a camera when I cannot see well enough to distinguish the settings? Since I cannot read the small numbers and icons without magnification, I have learned to set up the camera beforehand the way I think I will want it—to make the colors vivid and the outlines sharp—adjusting the exposure compensation, underexposing to bring out the colors. I will have to hold the camera very still, hold my breath, which I only sometimes remember to do. I don't want those vivid colors to be blurry. I will then use the telephoto lens, moving it closer in to limit the amount of light coming through. Admitting less light will produce richer colors, but less of a total vista. I tend to focus in closely most of the time so that, in the end, I can distinguish an object as if it were right in front of me, so it will make more sense to me and create a better picture. Where someone with better sight might see the tiny focus points, using them to adjust the exposure more precisely, I simply zoom in until the sunrise colors become dramatic. Then I readjust the composition and try to snap the shot quickly before the camera makes up its mind to reread the light and change the settings. I try to do this with some thought, but rapidly so that I will get a picture that is both vibrant in color and balanced and interesting in design before the shutter clicks.

Back at the house later in the day, I put my pictures into my laptop and study them, looking for the exposure settings and the focus points so that I can learn from them and take better pictures next time. I sit at my computer, with my eyes close to the screen, trying to see the small print that tells me what my settings were— minus .3 at 185 mm, ISO 800, and so forth. I have the computer— with its synthesized voice and text-to-speech software—read these settings aloud to me at the same time as I peer at them. Where was the main focus point? I strain to see it. It is easier to see the complete image than all these small details. The image now large and vivid on my screen shows the huge pink cloud that hung over the house this morning when I snapped the shot. It looks like a nice pink cloud, but fuzzy. Here's a photo that is totally red in the background—a small piece of red-hot sky magnified with bare tree branches in the foreground. On one branch, Hannah has pointed out to me, a tiny bird was silhouetted in black against the red sky, perched on a branch also silhouetted in black, enjoying the early dawn before everyone was up—before the light, before the noise, the dust of cars and road—while a woman with a camera squinted into the dark, trying to see and not to fall as she took a step closer to the sky, to the redness in the distance behind the trees and over the hills, toward a mountainside not too far off—the tree-covered cliffs of the Gila wilderness.

As I stepped forward, cane outstretched, I suddenly heard the sound of trampling hoofs and a snort. "Oh, no!" I thought, I had lost my way on the road, so eager was I to see the sky. I had walked toward it and was now in a tangle of low scrub. I heard another snort, and back and forth went those hoofs. I held my camera close, protecting it, and probed ahead with my cane. It got stuck in a bush. I shook it loose and headed for the opposite side of the road, wanting not to be trampled or bitten. I thought either these were deer or javelinas from the forest, or that I had stepped into a horse enclosure on someone's property while thinking I was still on the road. I could see nothing in the dark. Only later on my way back, when it was finally light enough for me to see the ground, did I find a mule trotting back and forth on the other side of a barbed wire fence. She was lit from behind, the sun coming through her whiskers, looking straight at me, her mouth open with a snort, wanting a treat. I raised my camera and took her picture. I have several photos of that neighbor's mule. I show these to other people and the image is not as meaningful to them as it is to me—for it stands for my fears in the dark and of what I don't see. And it stands for that light that I seek out again and again. Why do I try so hard to see? Why not give up? But then I would be giving up on my life, I feel. My life did not change when I became blind, or as I become more blind.

And yet it does. It becomes more complex. I often feel frustrated and incompetent when I cannot move quickly; when I bump into things I don't see; when I must reread my writing over and over by listening to it rather than scanning it with my eyes; when I peer at objects long and hard and still I miss parts of them; when I must wait for buses and for rides. Often, "I cannot" is the first thing that comes to my mind. And then I must remind myself, "I can." I can do this; I can move around, accomplish my tasks; I can "see" in the ways that are necessary for me. I am not damaged goods, a failed person, someone whom life is passing by. With my careful movements and my limited sight, this *is* my life. I can create something out of the confusion around me, use my ingenuity.

Back when I was first losing my eyesight in a way that affected my mobility, I was driving one morning in that beautiful dark before sunrise to the desert wildlife refuge Hannah and I often visit when, like this morning in the mountains, I was struck by how hard it was for me to see the ground. In that case, it was the black asphalt road as I drove toward the refuge and then the dirt road within it, which was even harder to see because the earth, more than the asphalt, absorbed the light. In the darkness, I strained to see the edges of the road to maintain my route. At one point soon after I had started out, I turned into someone's yard by accident and almost hit their house; luckily, a chain link fence stopped me. That same morning, I missed my turn onto the refuge, went past it on the asphalt road, and then I had to turn the car around to come back and find my exit. But it was so dark and my eyesight so poor that I could not see the edges of the road to make my U-turn. I kept getting out of the car, looking at the ground—putting my head down close to it—to find out exactly where it was and where the edges were—then getting back in the car, turning a bit, getting out, looking down, getting in and finally completing the turn. That was the way I did it then. I trusted putting my eyes up close to things and making my way on foot more than when driving the car. Now that I no longer drive, my way on foot is questionable. What will disappear next?

That morning in Pinos Altos as I ran from the mule, I had not asked Hannah to come with me to guide me to see the sky. I wanted to find my way alone in the dark to take my pictures and experience the excitement of the dawn. I also wanted to reach the edge of a hillside not far off to view the sunrise colors from a different angle, but I could not take those extra steps. I thought I should have scouted out my route in more detail beforehand to identify which ruts to notice and when to make my turns. Then I might not have frightened the mule who scared me, and I might have gone further on the road. But it is hard not to get lost in the darkness. Even in very familiar places, and even with Teela leading me, I sometimes become lost. I used to like being lost, glad for the surprises, the new scenes, the sense of adventure in following where a road might take me. But getting lost while blind feels more dangerous—will I ever be found, will I be safe? I so want to step toward the sky, the dream, the future, the excitement, the new. Yet I often feel daunted by the limitations in my mobility. Where are my new experiences to come from if I cannot move more freely and arrive at different angles from which I might see? Still I take pleasure in what comes.

I enjoyed my views of the sunrise colors this morning, deepened and framed through my lens. The colors were all the more meaningful to me because my blindness usually washes out colors, making them seem dim and far off. But with the darkness in the background, with the magnification of the camera, focusing in on the spot of richest hue, I was overwhelmed with the beauty of what

I could see. I felt I was capturing the vividness within the oranges, the reds. I was in touch with the essence of something quickly gone. I walked back to the house where we were staying, camera in hand, the sky a bit lighter, seeing the ground more clearly now. I felt shocked that it was there—so easy to make out. The ground of this dirt road was plain compared with the prior light show overhead. It looked solid. It was hard to imagine I had ever lost my way upon it. When Hannah woke up, I showed her my pictures of the dramatic colors, the tree branches, the dark shapes of houses in the early dawn, the golden reflections everywhere when the first light after sunrise illumined wooden and adobe homes and juniper trees. Hannah dutifully marveled at what I had taken, making me feel that my finds, my adventures, were worthwhile—my small glimpses of something special.

That winter as Hannah, Teela, and I traveled in the New Mexico countryside, not only did my trouble seeing the ground repeatedly surprise me, but Hannah had a shoulder injury, which caused her much pain when opening the car door. I would get out of the car each time we stopped, go around to her side, and open the door for her so she could get out without straining her left shoulder. When getting in the car, too, I would first close her door for her so she would not have to reach over. Her shoulder was so painful that even driving in the car—the jostling and vibration of it against her seat belt constraint—hurt her. Here we were, I thought: I couldn't see well, so Hannah had to drive us, and each time we stopped, I got out and went around and opened the door for her because her shoulder hurt. Teela sat on the back seat peering out at me as I moved slowly, touching the body of the car and then the hood as I circled, wanting not to trip on an invisible snag at my feet. Hannah and I were an odd couple, I thought, caring for each other in this way. Sometimes it was hard because Hannah would be irritable because of her shoulder and I would be irritable because of my frustration about my eyes. But we did okay. I was proud of us. I simply had to suspend an image I kept having that it should not be like this. Hannah should be able to drive without pain. I should be able to drive, and to walk without calculating every step.

One day when we had driven into a local town so Hannah could use the therapeutic pool in a health center to do exercises for her shoulder, I had planned to walk to a Mexican restaurant while waiting for her. As Teela and I headed over, I soon realized this was going to be harder than I thought. Walking through the parking lots that lay between the health center and the restaurant, I quickly stumbled and became afraid. There were many irregularities in the asphalt and no straight lines for Teela to follow in guiding me, and the sun was hazy and bright. The glare from the sun, combined with my lack of depth perception, made the ground look like a shimmering black blur. I urged Teela to follow an adjacent sidewalk for a while, but it ran out, and it, too, was cracked and irregular in places. I was trying to walk where people don't usually walk—through parking lots to buildings they usually drive to. Cars might come fast through the parking lots and not expect to see us. One could hit us. It felt dangerous and I was afraid. Teela and I made it to the restaurant and back, but it was not something I would do again. This was not the early morning darkness of a dirt road in Pinos Altos, but the light of a busy town in midday. Still the ground felt almost equally undecipherable. The sun was bright, the sky clear but for high white clouds. I could see that beautiful sky, yet I could not see the ground. That is something I always need to remember. What is it? Is it that I should look to the sky when the ground is cracked and uneven? Look up and see the clouds, the light, the new excitement. But don't forget the ground. Feel it with your toes; let Teela show it to you; use your cane; walk slowly. Don't worry about what other people will think. That is easy to say, harder to incorporate within myself, for the opposites often don't mix, and the light in the sky makes it seem as if the ground should be easy to know, when, in fact, it takes much concentration to move about, to find my way. If I do not focus intently on the ground, I may trip, but if I focus too much and don't look up, I will miss the colors changing in the sky.

This past winter on our trip to New Mexico, we returned to Pinos Altos, and when I went outside before sunrise the first morning, it had snowed. Magically, the ground was white, reflecting what little light was in the sky. I was overjoyed! I could see it. I knew, however, that I could not see the actual ground beneath the snow. That still had ruts; there might be ice. There were so many ways to fall. I had not taken Teela with me. I did not want her standing out in the snow getting icy feet. So here I was again in the dark alone, unsure of my footsteps, yet looking to the sky. The white snow on everything gleamed. The sky this morning was not as colorful as it had been the year before, because it was a snow sky—overcast with moisture—but it was beautiful—strangely eerie. Christmas lights hung on houses, cars and rooftops were capped with snow, tree branches laden—it was a wonderland for me. I was eager to take pictures and bring them back inside, and worried about my camera getting wet from the snow. But it worked out. My pictures showed the snow gray-white in the darkness, thick on houses, trees, and the road, the more austere surroundings softly lit. All during that trip as we rode around, the mountains and fields in the distance were covered with white, making only the prominent shapes of trees, buildings, and land forms stand out. It was all in relief, a gift to the unsighted. The ground was covered with an iridescent glow, even the cars looked nice. Everywhere we went, the landscape was decked out with white robes or with a thin veneer of white. This year, Hannah no longer had a shoulder injury, so her driving was more relaxed. Teela played in the snow, bounding gleefully through the drifts. A photo I have of her sunlit in the snow is one of my favorites of all time. Hannah built a snow person that turned into a lamb. We enjoyed our time, the moveable home of our car, the houses in which we stayed. I enjoyed the cold, which made our fires indoors all the warmer. One year there was darkness, and now there was light, as if the sky had hit the ground—the big expanses made easy to see and clean—a new treat for the eyes, even my failing ones.

I am looking forward to our next winter's trip to the desert when I will see again a landscape I miss. Will I see colors; will there be snow? Will Teela be with me? Will she be retired yet? Will I be willing to ask Hannah to drive me on some of those early mornings when I have previously gone out alone? I might then go farther and see the sky from different angles. It's hard to be mobile, I often feel, especially with all the dangers around—falling in ruts, being hit by a car, startling mules, getting lost. But my mobility is important, the mobility in my mind—the flexibility, adaptability. Amidst all the uncertainties I feel as what I saw yesterday slips away and as I seek not to let my limitations diminish me, I know that a central element for me is taking care—of Teela, of Hannah, and of myself. And it's letting Hannah take care of me—feeling her care in her driving me to see the sights, her appreciation of my finds—as we share the pleasures, the relaxation, the willingness to take it on, as Hannah helps me see the ground and I bring home pieces of the sky.

August 2012

Part III

Weathering Life's Losses

EIGHT

On a Distant Hillside

My mother died three and-a-half weeks ago, on Tuesday, December 8, at 1:43 p.m. eastern time. December is usually my month since it is the month of my birthday, December 28. Now it is also the month of my mother's death. In late September when I visited my mother, she had felt she was in good health, although she was easily short of breath. Ten weeks later, she was gone. My sister called me the week before. "Mother is dying," she said full of tears. "If you want to see her, you had better come back now." Teela and I got on a plane. My sister and her husband picked us up at the Philadelphia airport, bringing a dog food bowl for Teela and a sandwich for me, and we drove up to Connecticut to the assisted living residence where my mother was now in the nursing unit of the complex.

As I stepped into the room where she lay on her back in a single bed, I bent over to give her a kiss. "I'm glad you're here," she said warmly and graciously, her voice musical, as it has always been. Earlier in the week, when I spoke with my mother on the phone and told her I would be arriving in two days, she had said, "I guess I'll keep eating then." She was preparing to die. That was a concept hard for me to understand, for I so wanted her to live.

I spent that next weekend visiting with my mother, sitting with her before her death, telling her I loved her, looking out for her care, sleeping on the couch back in her apartment, which, with her gone, seemed oddly vacant, although it was filled with my sister, her husband, her three grown daughters, with me and Teela, and with my sister's oldest daughter's small dog. But my mother was not there. Her furniture lay around us, reflecting her careful way of setting things out: a newspaper she had been reading was still on the stool beside her chair, the crossword puzzle incompletely finished; food on the kitchen counters seemed left as if she had just stepped out for a short while. But she would not be coming back. She could no longer walk and was more comfortable in the other wing of the residence, receiving nursing care, breathing with supplemental oxygen.

That weekend as I sat with her in her nursing home room, Teela quietly lying on the floor by my side, an oxygen mask sometimes totally covered my mother's nose and mouth, making it hard for me to understand her words. But when she breathed through a smaller oxygen tube placed beneath her nose, I could hear her more clearly. She was definite in her wishes. "I want to die today," she told the hospice evaluator who came to review her condition on Saturday. "Can you give me something?"

"We can't legally do that," the hospice representative said. "But we can make you more comfortable." The woman then came out to the lounge nearby where my sister Kathe, her daughters, and I sat around a table. She advised us that we should each tell my mother it was all right with us that she "let go." Kathe's daughters dutifully agreed, but it was not all right with me. I told them I did not want my mother to die, so I could not tell her that, but that I wouldn't argue with her either. I would tell her I loved her and that she should have what she needed, which is what I did that weekend.

I love my mother and I have always loved her. I love her all the more now that she is gone. However, I also feel a certain block within myself, a wall, a sense that I do not have the proper feelings with regard to her death. I am overwhelmingly sad for her. I did not want her to die. I felt she died prematurely, although she was eigty-seven, that she should have lived another few years. But the doctors did not know how to rid her system of accumulated fluid in her lungs. In my mind, it is unbelievable that the medical system could not do more for my mother. I feel that the medical world failed her, and that is my most difficult thought to tolerate. My mother's brother, who is a doctor, told me one day as we stood in the hallway beside her room that she was given a medication for heart fibrillations two years earlier, after her heart valve operation, and that medication may have had the side effect of damaging the blood vessels in her lungs. Thus they could not do their job. Her stressed heart developed hypertension. The right side of it, becoming weakened, could not pump the fluids out from her system in the end. Finally, my mother's lungs filled up with fluid and she stopped breathing.

My sister was with her when she died. I left two days before, on Sunday. She died Tuesday afternoon. Kathe called me right afterward. "Mother died," she said. "Damn," I said. "How long ago?" "One minute."

My sister explained further: "The aide called me over. I had just stepped toward the dresser. I stood with Mother and told her I loved her and that she was the best mother in the world, and she stopped breathing."

I would not have said my mother was the best mother in the world, but she was *my* mother. She was a unique person, not always easy on those around her, volatile, tall, intelligent, intuitive, proud in how she carried herself, caring of others, superior in many ways, a person I have always not only looked up to, but looked out for. As kids, we used to hang around my mother, or I did, watching her carefully, watching out for her to make sure she was okay, still with us, still functioning as our mother. She moved through the world fiercely self-reliant, yet at the same time conveying a need for our care.

In the weeks immediately before my mother died, I often spoke with her on the phone, far more often than was usual for us. We ended each call by saying, "Love you," or "I love you." My mother did not normally say that to me, and I almost never said it to her. But now we both did, quickly and meaningfully. My mother was in the nursing unit by that time. Her doctors were trying to rid her system of the fluids, but it was not going well. My mother's primary physician spoke with me several times to keep me updated. Initially, he thought she would be able to return to her apartment and explained to me that hers was not an end-of-life situation. Before I understood it, however, my mother understood that her condition was not going to improve. At one point on the phone, she reprimanded me for my ignorance, telling me I had my "head in the clouds" and that I did not know anything. I told her I wanted to hope for the best, and why couldn't she do that too? She might get better. But she turned out to be right and I was wrong. I have often felt that my mother is right and that I must be wrong. This is, in part, because my mother is so smart—or she was—intensely intelligent, astute, quick-minded. She seemed to know everything, and she tended always to insist on her stance, as if her life depended on it, often criticizing or cutting down the opposition. Often she would strike out at me or in my direction with her words or gestures. Because of that, it has been hard for me to feel I am right, to trust my judgment, to feel I can take care of myself, that my impulses are good.

My mother's habits of hostility toward me persisted through to the time of her death. They were noticeable to me during my visit—small ways of striking out that did not hurt me as much as they reminded me that she was still my mother, her personality intact. At the same time, her reprimands, criticisms, and deliberate silences affirmed something within me, took me off the hook, made me feel it was okay to leave her.

My mother's repeated hostile gestures were perhaps characteristic of a person's frustrations with being sick or dying, but also characteristic of my mother's particular relationship with me. For example, one morning when I arrived in her room to greet my mother and bent over to give her a kiss on her forehead, I said, "I love you," and asked how she was. "Back off," she belted out to me. Then she turned to my sister, who was standing by my side, and began talking softly with her. I felt, right then, that my mother did not trust me, but I was glad that she trusted Kathe, who has long befriended her and helped her through hard times. Unlike me, my sister does not confront my mother, or differ with her directly. She keeps quiet, goes along, and eases them both through any difficulty. She does what my mother wants and takes care of her needs. I felt it was fortunate that my mother had my sister, especially now.

Another time when I greeted my mother—"I'm here, how are you?" I said, taking my seat beside her bed, settling Teela next to me. "Get that dog out of here," my mother commanded. "People can't move around." I hurriedly took Teela to the opposite end of the room, then out into the hall. It was understandable, I thought, a big dog in a small nursing home room. Yet there was a disregard in my mother's tone, a harshness. I felt put at a distance and hurt that I could offer neither my dog nor myself as a comfort. I did bring Teela back with me after that when I went in to visit my mother, since I needed her there for myself, but I was careful to keep her out of the way.

While we were at my mother's bedside that weekend, my sister would sometimes hold up for my mother a photograph album with pictures from my family's past—of my mother and father when young, of my parents with us as kids, of my mother with my sister's three daughters. My mother would then comment on the photos. She seemed pleased to see them. "We were a good-looking couple," she said of one of her with my father. "That's when we were about to tell our parents we were going to get married."

Often when I sat next to my mother, it was in silence, keeping her company. At first, I tried to fill the blank spaces with talk, idle chatter about myself or her, bringing her up to date. Then my sister's husband came back to my mother's apartment and told me, "Don't talk when you're there. She wants quiet."

"Okay," I said, but I felt hurt. I was doing something for my mother that she could not now do—carrying on with life—and I was supposed to stop. I did not understand why. Hannah suggested later on the phone: "She's competitive with you. When you talk, it's about you. Your mother wants to be the center of attention. It's always been like that."

Sometimes when I sat with her, I touched my mother's hand or put my hand lightly on her right arm, which lay at her side near me. I wanted her to feel I was with her. The first time I did that, it seemed all right with her. She lay still, breathing in her oxygen. But the next time I touched her arm, she shook me off. She roused from her stillness to get rid of my hand, although I had thought it was gently placed. I pulled it back, but her gesture made me wonder if all my advances were so unwanted, if everything I did was just too much for her. Had it always been that way? I thought so. I did not want to be an unwanted weight, a burden, or an intrusion.

After that, when I sat with my mother and bent close to her head to tell her I loved her, and that she should tell us what she needed, I felt I was probably mumbling too many "sweet nothings" in her ear. And that now that she was incapacitated, she could not tell me so. I decided to do it anyway.

On one of those afternoons as Teela, Kathe, and I were sitting with her, my mother said something about my being bossy. I had just stood up and was moving toward the foot of her bed, and I did not understand the comment. It was not quite an insult. Just before, my mother had begun to speak to my sister and me about what needed to be done in the cemetery. I leaned close, listening as she spoke, and quickly reassured her that she need not worry. Kathe and I had taken care of it. It would all go smoothly, I told her. She could relax and focus on her comfort in the present. "There won't be many people there," she said.

"Of course there will be," I answered.

I think my sister wanted to hear more of what my mother was about to say concerning the cemetery. My stopping her may have been why my mother thought I was bossy. Later, my sister told me that my mother thought I always "solved things," and that this was a good trait. Maybe that is what I had done with regard to the cemetery. I only knew that I could not bear talking with my mother about her graveside while she was still alive.

A few times as I sat with my mother, when she needed to be attended to by the aides or nurses—for her bedding to be changed or her mouth to be swabbed with moisturizing fluid—when I volunteered to get an aide, or to help her in some way, she reprimanded me. "You don't know how things work here," she said. "You just don't know." I felt hurt that she did not trust me to help her, and also that she was telling me that I was not in charge, she was: she knew when to press the button for an aide, how long you waited. Still, I had that sense that she was unsatisfied with me, that I had failed her somehow.

On Saturday noon when my mother began eating what turned out to be her last meal, my sister sat beside her to help her. I took a seat in a chair at the foot of her bed, looking over toward my mother as she haltingly sampled the various foods on her tray, deciding that none of them tasted good enough to be worth eating further. I watched as she gently lifted a bowl of soup and then a glass of milk to her lips. She mostly drank the milk. I marveled internally that she could still drink milk, that it did not disagree with her as it did with me. My sister helped her lift the dishes. When my mother was finished with the meal, she looked down the length of the bed toward me. "I don't like you watching me eat," she said.

"I can go out," I offered and stood to leave.

"It's already done," she said.

"My vision is blurry, I didn't see you well." I came over and bent to be close to her, trying to improve the situation.

"I know that," my mother said very definitely, displaying her sense that it did not matter, I had already seen too much. I felt reprimanded. I felt that I should have known that she would not want me to watch her eat. Too much intimacy was involved perhaps. Or maybe she knew that I would want her to eat. Thus if she did not, she was doing something I did not want, something wrong: she was preparing to die. I think my mother knew I did not want her to die, and that this last struggle was one she was going to win. She would have it her way, die when she wanted to, even if her oldest daughter would have had it all work out differently.

On one of those last times when I was with my mother, sitting beside her, my head bent close to listen to her softly spoken words, I heard her say, "I never expected this." I thought she was then going to tell me that she never expected to be laid up as an invalid in a hospice bed so soon. "The tenderness," she whispered. "I never expected the tenderness, the feeling from so many people. They really care. They gave a party for me." I heard her gently cry.

I felt, right then, that my mother felt that if she was going to die, this was the best way it could be. I also felt that she had in mind the care she received from the nursing staff—the aides, the nurses and doctors, the hospice people—on whom she knew she was dependent. I did not feel she was referring to care from me. Yet I also cared about her and I felt tender toward her, although I knew she was not dependent on me in the same way.

Before I left her on Sunday, I told my mother that she should be sure to keep telling the nursing staff what she needed so that she could have her needs met. I told her I loved her, and would always love her, and that I would keep her with me in good ways, that Kathe would still be there after I left, and that if she needed me, I could come back. She lay still and did not say anything. Perhaps she did not hear me, maybe she did. I will never know. I think that even if she heard me, my mother was not going to respond, for we did not have that kind of relationship. If I needed a response from her right at the moment, my mother would, as a rule, withhold it—wanting, perhaps, not to be controlled by a willful first child—and simply because she was dying now, it did not change what always was. I kissed my mother on her forehead, my beautiful mother, and I left her.

In the hallway outside her room, I sobbed. My sister came and put her arms around me. Her daughter Julia handed me two tissues. My tears felt relieving, real, cool, like water from a fresh shower.

I was raised by my mother to be generous, to extend myself to others in my own way. I think that, in her way, my mother was generous to me. She did not throw me out of her nursing home room, or refuse to see me, or hurl a plate, as she had often done in my childhood when she became angry or frustrated beyond cause. She did not refuse me simply because I had left her so many years ago—moved away, far away to California, as soon as I could, to enter graduate school, then to live there permanently. Back then, California was a greater distance from the East than it is now. After I left, I came back to visit my parents infrequently and never stayed long enough. "I think your mother feels abandoned by you," Hannah told me on one of our calls. But though I left my mother, I did not cut all ties with her, nor she with me. We always sought connection.

My sister's husband and her daughter Julia drove Teela and me to the Philadelphia airport Sunday afternoon, where they dropped us off on their way back to Wilmington, Delaware, where they live. As Teela and I sat in the airport, I called my mother's sister, who lives in Maine, to tell her how my mother was doing. Kathe stayed on in Connecticut with my mother, unsure how long she would be there, taking it day to day. By then, my mother was at ease, made comfortable by the medicines given to her to relieve any pain or emotional distress she might feel. She had round-the-clock individual care. She was lying still, resting, quiet, dying in the way she wanted. My sister was with her. She and I had thought that my mother might live until the next weekend, but she died sooner than we expected.

I arrived home late Sunday night and soon began packing for a trip to New Mexico that I had long planned that would take me to places always a haven for me. Three days later, Hannah, Teela, and I boarded an airplane and took off for the desert. Before I left the East Coast, my sister and I had discussed what we would do after our mother died. We had planned that Kathe would take care of the cemetery by herself, with the support of her family, and that a memorial could wait until my return in two weeks. But plans change. Late the afternoon before I left for the desert, my sister called to tell me there would be a ceremony on the upcoming Sunday in the New Haven Jewish cemetery, where my father and brother were also buried. She had spoken with the rabbi and that was when he could do it. She was also planning a gathering at my mother's residence for after the cemetery for people from the residence who could not make it out. She asked if I would be there.

"I'll think about it," I said, not wanting to be too abrupt in my answer. After considering, I called her back. "I want to go on my trip," I told her. I wished to say that my mother would have wanted me to go to New Mexico—and not be there when her ashes were lowered into the ground—but, of course, these were my wishes, not hers. I wanted to take my trip, and I did not want my mother to stop me, even with her death. I did not want her ruining my life or my happiness, an impulse I have probably had since young and long cultured within myself—unaware, much of the time, of the importance of it. This is an impulse I draw upon daily as I battle, within myself, the negatives, the self-criticisms and self-doubts instilled, in part, by my relationship with my mother, internalizations of her striking out.

When I told my sister I would not be coming back for the service at the cemetery, she paused on the phone. I could feel she wanted me there, and I understood that taking care of these things sooner was best, though I still felt a pull to go on my trip. "My girls are very traditional," my sister said, "they'll feel okay about your not being there if I'm okay with it, but they won't really understand."

I then volunteered to call and speak with my nieces the night before the cemetery service: "I'll explain and let them know how much I will be there with them in spirit."

When we arrived in the desert, I immediately took comfort from the countryside—the open landscape, the big sky, the subtle colors, even the bare trees. I felt grateful for everything I saw, felt, and ate—for the winter, the warmth indoors, the bird refuge we visited, although there were few birds. I was happy to be on my trip and surprised by how much my surroundings pleased me. It took no effort to be pleased, and usually adjusting to a new place takes much effort on my part.

Each day, I spoke with my sister on the phone. She had written an obituary for the paper and a moving remembrance of my mother to read at the ceremonies. I wrote and sent her a remembrance of mine to read as well. The day of the cemetery service was soon changed to Monday, in the morning, because the undertaker told my sister that Sunday afternoon in winter back East would be dark and depressing. Sunday night, I called and spoke with my sister's daughters and explained and apologized. I thought of telling them that my mother would have wanted me to take my trip, but it wasn't true, so I told them I had a plan. At the same time as they would be in the Mishkan Israel cemetery in New Haven, I would be in a cemetery in New Mexico also observing my mother's death. I would be far away, but I hoped this parallel observance would make me feel closer.

Within myself, however, I felt that my absence was inexcusable. How could I not be at my mother's graveside when she was laid to rest? Still, I liked my plan. Hannah, Teela, and I would be going to a graveyard in the rural farming area where we were staying and would be there exactly when Kathe and her family convened in the cemetery back East. We had, the day before, scouted out two nearby cemeteries and picked the smaller one—located on a gentle hillside in a stretch of desert open to the sun and sky with a broad view of surrounding mountains. The small town the cemetery served had burned to the ground twenty years before, but the cemetery had survived. When we visited it to take a first look, I had walked around on the packed tan earth made hard and smooth by recent rains, and I had felt an openness among the scattered graves. Some of them were marked by stone plaques, others by simple wooden crosses. Hannah and I looked for Jewish graves but found none, for this was an old Hispanic Catholic cemetery. The names here were Padilla, Gutierrez, Flores. Not Cahn, Lipofsky, or Casher—the names from my extended family. It was a stretch to honor an Eastern Jewish woman in a Western Catholic graveyard, but it was a nice cemetery. Many of the graves were carefully decorated with flowers. Only when I bent to touch the flowers did I realize that they were made either of cloth or plastic, they looked so real.

After opening the gate to the cemetery, I had quickly begun looking for a worthy grave. I wanted to find the gravestone of a woman who had died to whom I could bring flowers on the day of my mother's ceremony back East. Teela led as Hannah and I climbed the hillside, exploring among the stones and crosses until, in the upper right-hand corner, I found her—sitting apart, her grave marked by an upright plaque that held the words, "Beloved Mother." I felt in luck, remembering that my sister and I had decided to put "Beloved" on my mother's stone. In full the inscription on the plaque before me read: "Francisca T. Saavedra, Beloved Mother, 1877–1940." I looked closely at her stone and thought that Francisca might like some flowers. Maybe she had no children around now to take care of her.

After walking farther through the small, sun-baked cemetery, we left, planning to return Monday morning. Hannah and I then searched in a nearby town for flowers to bring to Francisca's grave—not plastic or cloth flowers, but real ones, the kind my mother would like. The best flowers in town were in the supermarket, where, at first, I reached for a pot of bright red poinsettias, bold in color and full of life. But these were Christmas flowers. Too Christian, Hannah and I both knew. It was bad enough that we would be in a Catholic cemetery, not a Jewish one. Luckily, nearby stood a large bunch of white chrysanthemums mixed with green junipers. My mother especially prized chrysanthemums. She had a large picture of a cluster of white chrysanthemums hanging on her living room wall, surrounded by a yellow background. She felt the picture was cheerful. When she moved to her nursing home room, she had her chrysanthemum picture brought over, where it hung on the wall opposite her bed, brightening her day. When I arrived, I saw it there as familiar to me as my mother.

I snatched up the lovely bunch of white chrysanthemums in the market and handed them to Hannah. Driving home to our bed and breakfast, I told her I thought I would put my mother's flowers out in a vase on the dining room table for people to appreciate before we took them to the cemetery, since there they would quickly dry up and blow away.

"I don't know if that's a good idea," Hannah said. "People will wonder why you're not back there."

I put the flowers out, not wanting to feel ashamed. Sunday night, I described them to my sister's daughters: "The other graves have plastic or cloth flowers, but you know your grandmother. She would want the flowers to be real." Each daughter agreed. I could hear their smiles through the phone and it seemed to ease things. If I was not there, if the cemetery was Catholic not Jewish, at least the flowers would be real.

The next morning as a group of family and friends gathered in the Mishkan Israel Jewish cemetery in Connecticut, Hannah, Teela, and I gathered in the San Pedro Catholic cemetery in New Mexico, on a hillside under a white, weathering sky, to honor the memory of my mother. At the cemetery in New Haven, quite a few other people were present in addition to my sister's family. Kathe read the obituary she had written and both her remembrance and mine. My mother's brother spoke. My mother's sister called in from Maine and participated on a speakerphone. The rabbi spoke. A box of my mother's ashes was lowered into the ground. At the same time, I knelt by the grave of another "beloved mother" out on a windswept plain, on a hillside beneath a shining sky, with snow-covered mountain peaks in the distance, my cherished guide dog by my side. Emotion in her voice, Hannah stood nearby and said Kaddish, the Jewish prayer for the dead taking the loved one back into the kingdom of God.

Kneeling by Francisca's grave, I then said some words of love for my mother that were quickly swept away by the desert winds as tears came to my eyes. I asked Hannah to take a video of our small ceremony to send back to my sister and her family to make my absence seem more present. On the video, as I placed the flowers by the grave, my words are only faintly audible—"Mother." "Surrounded by." I think having that video is mostly important for me, although we took it for others. It makes me feel less absent, more like I was honoring my mother even if far away.

When I was back East before my mother died, my sister and I had discussed what we would like to put on her gravestone. We debated and then decided on, "Rhoda Cahn, Beloved, 1922–2009." On Francisca Saavedra's stone, it said, "Beloved Mother," but simply "Beloved" seemed best for my mother. I thought she was probably beloved by other people than us. I also thought it was a good thing to recognize that a person could be loved despite difficulties.

Standing now in the San Pedro cemetery, surrounded by mountains and yellowing plains—caught in the winds between a vast stretch of desert five miles to the east, where once the first atomic bomb had been set off, and to the west, across the Rio Grande, a marshland where a sequestered wildlife refuge lay—I felt lucky to have found the grave of another "beloved mother." Where, at first, I had looked for the grave of a Jewish woman but found that not a realistic possibility here, where the graves read, "Here lies Cowboy," or "Recuerdo de Su Familia," I had soon found that lone stone for "Francisca T. Saavedra." Not Rhoda Cahn, or Rhoda Lipofsky Cahn, but the word "beloved" was there and both were mothers. I had begun to feel fond of Francisca Saavedra. I wondered what her life had been like, where her descendants were, and why she was so alone in this cemetery.

I took a picture of her stone with my good camera. The first day we visited, I had taken a picture of her stone bathed in golden sunlight. Today the sky was overcast so the light was different, but the inscription was clear. Hannah took several photos of Teela and me next to the stone with the white chrysanthemums standing in a bunch up against it. We had placed them to one side in order not to obscure the writing. I wanted to send these pictures to my sister, to keep them for myself. We had also put two small rocks on top of Francisca's gravestone, following the Jewish tradition of adding to the monument, placing the stones to indicate that someone has come to visit, that the deceased has not been forgotten. Hannah found the small stones on the ground when we first entered the cemetery. They appear in all the photos we took and in the video— sitting atop Francisca's square, gray plaque, white flowers decorating its front—this offering from afar to my sister and her family, to my mother and to another now long gone woman to make it seem not as incongruous as it might that I was not back there in the East with my mother's ashes, but here out under the Western desert sky.

I did not plan my words at Francisca's grave. I simply said some of the things I had told my mother back when I last visited with her—about how I loved her and always would. I did not plan my words because I didn't think, at the time, that I needed a ceremony or a speech. I was doing this gesture for others, to make up for my absence. Maybe I did not need a ceremony, maybe I did. Maybe I needed a ceremony not back there, but far away, off by myself in my world. I wondered if my mother would have liked it here, liked this windswept hillside, this open desert. She liked the ocean more, I thought, a familiar landscape from her childhood. But sometimes I thought she would like the desert, the spareness of it, the calming sense of order. She liked my photographs of mountains when I had showed them to her on my visit two months before. Those pictures showed vast open stretches of desert with a few mountain ranges at the borders, taken down in the very south near Mexico. My mother would not like the wind and cold here today, I thought, but she would like the peacefulness.

As I knelt beside Francisca's grave, I told my mother that I would keep her with me in good ways. Telling her that was hard for me to say, as it had been when I said it to her back in her nursing home room. For keeping my mother with me in positive ways too easily recalls the negatives for me, the self-undermining voices that I must fight. Yet that is what I felt I needed to say. As I spoke, wind blowing, Hannah filming with our tiny snapshot camera, Teela beside me alertly watching the flowers and the surrounding plains for prey, I motioned with my hands to indicate the landscape for my sister, describing the mountains and the cemetery, the beauty of the scene, the remembering of my mother, keeping her with me. In the video I hear again the wind; see the grave, the flowers, Francisca, Teela, myself; feel Hannah nearby; hear words about a Jewish mother far, far away.

After our ceremony, Hannah went back to the car to stay warm, taking Teela with her. I checked that the chrysanthemums still stood firmly up against Francisca's grave, the two stones on top, the flower stems carefully wrapped in a plastic bag and stuck deeply into the earth to keep them from drying out. Hannah had pushed a larger rock against the stalks to hold the flowers upright. It was easier to leave a grave decorated by flowers.

I am not sure my mother ever would have understood why I chose this graveyard and ceremony. Like my sister's daughters, she was, at heart, traditional. Hannah, too, is traditional, especially with regard to Jewish customs, so, fortunately, she knew enough of the Kaddish and that we had to place the stones. I was grateful that she was willing to come to this cemetery with me, since honoring my mother here was not the type of observance she would have chosen. But, knowing my needs, she did it for me.

With Hannah and Teela safely in the car, I spent the next half hour walking around the small San Pedro cemetery taking pictures with my camera, making the ground dusty from my footsteps, visiting almost every grave. I took some pictures I thought my sister would like, I took some searching for my mother, and for what I thought she would like. Maybe she would like that little sanctuary down the hill in the lower left corner of the cemetery, where two tall pines towered protectively over a plot with a central open stony area. A bench was placed to the side of the open area for people to sit on while visiting their dead. The trees seemed regularly watered by runoff. The plot had a wire mesh fence around it to keep the rabbits out of some low-growing vegetation. The little sanctuary—green against the barren tan of the rest of the cemetery—held the graves of a husband and a wife, each marked with a cross. The tall trees above framed a view of a distant snow-covered mountain. My mother would like this place, I thought. I imagined her sitting on the bench beside me. We would look off into the distance and we would talk.

I then walked among the other plots—some with several family members buried together surrounded by black wrought iron fencing, the graves decorated with flowers or a picture of a saint. One gravestone had an American flag on one side of it, a bright yellow cloth sunflower glowing on the other. I took its picture. I took pictures of weathered wooden crosses, pictures of the mountains and the plains, none of my pictures doing the scene justice, but making it memorable, helping me to see it, to think of my mother, to honor the dead.

Half an hour passed quickly as I wandered the hillside, feeling the mounds of departed souls at my feet, the irregular ground, and then I went back to visit Francisca. I took several more pictures of her gravestone with the flowers in front of it. I even took one from behind the stone to capture what the view looking out from it was like, to see what Francisca, and my mother, now saw. That picture has the gravestone's blank gray back, the mountains it looks toward far ahead, and a hint of white chrysanthemums peeking out from the side.

When I was a young girl, I sometimes thought I wanted my mother to die, and that then other people would be nice to me. I would get the affection I needed. Now that my mother has died, I do not seem to want other people to come too close, or to be too nice. I fear the intimacies of others, just as, perhaps, my mother feared intimacy. I fear being disappointed by others, that their offers of solace, or sympathy, will prove hollow, or have no effect, feel like nothing much set against my loss. But more than that, I fear that others will expect me to grieve for my mother in ways I cannot. Mothers and motherhood are so overloaded with conventional sentiments suggesting goodness and apple pie, comfort and giving life. Yet I had a hostile mother, which requires that I take, and will probably always need to take, a great distance from her. At the same time, I replicate, within myself, many of her fears and self-doubts, her wishes, her resolute strengths, her needs for order and safety, her desires to take care, her striving for competence.

When I returned home from New Mexico and from my earlier trip back East, I saw flowers blooming in my yard—red fuchsia, yellow orchids, the beginnings of cineraria. Immediately, I thought of my mother, and I missed her with a start. I missed her more than

I had while away, for I used to tell her what was blooming in my backyard almost every time we spoke on the phone. We would begin our conversations by talking about the weather. She would say what her weather was, and I would say mine, and then I would tell her what was blooming in my yard. "The cineraria are about to come up," I'd say, knowing how much she liked these blue and purple tiny daisylike flowers. Then, of course, my mother would quickly change the subject to tell me about her flowers, or her friend's garden, or about her brother and how he was doing. She did not like the focus taken off herself for long.

The significance of cineraria between my mother and me suggests something further. In the East, according to my mother, cineraria must be grown in pots, and they are low growers. In California, as in my yard in San Francisco, they grow tall and like weeds, self-sowing in the cool winter dampness. When my mother and I speak of cineraria, as we did often in recent years, I think we are talking about the distance between us and about that time now long ago, although it seems like yesterday, when I left my mother and my father for the West Coast. Back then, when my parents visited me, we would marvel at how everything grew in California in all seasons, how exotic the plants were, and how different. You could walk out in shirtsleeves even in winter, the weather was always nice. People were different here, more relaxed.

New Mexico now has that exotic, special feel for me, but I know that California is the original faraway exotic place for my mother and me. It's the place I left her for, as I left her for lesbianism, for not having children, for not coming back often enough to visit or ever staying long enough. I did not stay with my mother through to the moment of her death. I did not want to see her die. I did not want that moment to stay with me forever. Neither did I want to see her ashes lowered into the ground. I did not want to feel that she had become a box of ashes, that she was that gone. I would have felt very angry had I been there, as I did when my father's ashes were lowered years before. I would have felt too distraught. I would have wanted to cry but been afraid to. I wanted to be spared all that.

The day I left my mother's bedside back in the nursing center, I felt relieved to cry. I have not cried since then, though I often feel a welling up, a few tears in private, an urge to cry.

I have a memory of my mother in her nursing home room lying on her back, breathing in the oxygen, her gray hair combed nicely, her face peaceful, her pose still. Then she rouses, talks about old times as my sister holds a photograph album up for her to see. She soon rests, lies back; she looks beautiful. I think I will always have an image of her in that bed—an image of stillness, gentleness, and beauty, and mixed with it those moments of striking out, of her quieting the outer world in which I sat. So I am glad that I also have another image following soon upon that one, an image of me with Hannah and Teela in the small San Pedro desert cemetery studying the grave of another "beloved mother," Francisca Saavedra, placing the white chrysanthemums and the two small stones, saying some words blown by the wind about how I loved my mother. She was Rhoda Adele Lipofsky Cahn, proud and self-possessed to the end. And I was on a distant hillside, caught up perhaps too much in a far off culture, but searching for her, for her happiness, for a sense of what she might like, and for a way to keep her with me like a precious gift, a diamond in the rough, a gleam, a ribbon of silver light.

January 2010

NINE

✦ ✦ ✦✦ ✦ ✦

My Mother's Bracelet

I AM WEARING MY MOTHER'S SILVER Navajo bracelet that dates from the 1930s. Shining brightly on my right wrist—a band of glowing silver decorated with two rows of delicate stamped feathers—this bracelet reminds me of my mother, making me happy. It makes me feel my mother is still with me, alive, watching over me protectively. When I look at it, I see her simple, elegant taste. I see how she looked when she wore it—thoughtful, beautiful, proud—how she appeared on the outside, though the internal picture will, of course, be more complex. My sister says this bracelet was given to my mother by my father's sister's mother-in-law, Florence, whom I never met. When my sister sent it to me four weeks ago, I put it on immediately and could not take it off. I slept wearing it that night. Each morning since then, I have put the bracelet on first thing when I dress, hoping it will bring me luck. When I look at it on my wrist during the day, I see my mother's arm merged with mine, and I feel comforted. I touch the shining silver surface, feel the indented shapes of the feathers. My fingers move down the two sloping sides. The bracelet is called "carinated" because it has a crown—a narrow ridge of gleaming silver on top from which the sides slope seamlessly down and away toward my wrist, forming a slim triangular shape. The feathers are arranged in groupings of two and three on each side, blackened gently to show their design. They suggest lightness, seem almost to fly away. Although slender, the bracelet is substantial in weight, but it rests easily on my wrist and feels surprisingly comfortable.

Wearing it causes me to think about my mother's death last December and about how it has affected me during this past year, but more than that, about how I wish it to affect me. I wish it to make me strong, to give me a new and untroubled life—one that shines like the ribbon of light on my wrist.

My mother's bracelet also draws me to see images of the cemetery in New Haven, Connecticut, where a new gravestone now sits marking her death. The gravestone stands three feet high, is three feet wide, has a Jewish star in the center on top and, beneath it, our family name, "Cahn," for this stone also marks the deaths of three other family members—my father, William, my brother, Daniel, and my father's sister, Minnie. Previously, they each had a small foot-stone—a square plaque in the ground. But my sister and I wanted to use the occasion of our mother's death to replace the old footstones with something upright that would do them better justice. The new gravestone for them has a shiny gray surface with a thin outline that frames the inscriptions. In the upper two corners are decorative floral designs. The stone sits on a dark granite base and looks dignified. The inscriptions my sister and I decided upon are carved beneath the family name, under the Jewish star. First is the one for my father, "William Cahn, Beloved Husband, Father, Writer, 1912–1976." Beneath his is my mother's name, "Rhoda Lipofsky Cahn, Beloved Wife, Mother, 1922–2009." My brother's inscription, "Daniel Cahn, Son, 1953–1985," appears in the lower left corner. In the lower right is my father's sister, "Minnie Cahn Wasserman, 1909–1994." My sister, Kathe, and I wanted the inscriptions to tell a story, even if brief, about how these people were related.

The gravestone honoring them was set in place only a month and a half ago. I have not yet visited it, since I have not been back East since visiting my mother the weekend before she died. But my sister has visited—she went there three days ago—and she has sent me photos. In them, the stately gravestone sits in the sun, its face glowing golden-gray, suggesting our family. In one of the pictures, my sister stands behind the gravestone to show me its height by comparison with hers. In another, she walks up to it with her new small puppy, Jazz, to show me how her puppy has grown, and to have the puppy meet Mother. My sister and I talk about her new puppy in each of our phone conversations recently in the same way we used to talk about our mother. "How is she doing? What can we do to help her? What has that puppy done now?" The focus gives us something in common to talk and care about now that our mother is gone.

In looking at the photos my sister sent, I noticed that the old footstones were still in the ground near the new gravestone. They are overgrown with grass. I have to call the monument company to ask that the footstone for my father be removed because it says, "U.S. Army, World War II," since the army paid for it, but my father was a pacifist. He would not like the association with violence. My mother must have been so distressed when he died that she let the army take care of it. The footstones for Danny and Minnie can stay. They look picturesque overgrown with the dry winter grass. I think my mother would like the new gravestone because she is there with her loved ones. She would like the smooth surface, the Jewish star, the fact that it is in the Mishkan Israel cemetery, the substantial size, but probably not the flowers carved in the upper corners—they would seem to her too frilly. My mother is the woman of the simple Navajo bracelet. However, I think she would agree to let the flowers stand.

When my sister and I initially envisioned a gravestone for my mother, we planned to replace the old footstones with four separate upright headstones. I volunteered to be in charge of making the arrangements since I had been absent at the service at the cemetery last year. I called, first, the funeral home director to ask his advice about alternatives. He immediately suggested having one monument for all four family members. "They were cremated," he said, explaining the basics to me. "You have two plots and four people. They are actually now all in one plot. The other one is empty." He paused, leaving a silence, waiting, I felt, for me to respond, as if he expected my sister and me to keep the second plot empty until one day we would rest there.

"We won't be using the other one," I said. "I'd like to put the monument over both plots."

He then suggested inscribing one name in each of the four corners on the stone, gave me a price, and referred me to a local monument company run by two brothers who were familiar with the cemetery. The brother I spoke with at Spencer Monument agreed that a common headstone was a good idea and sent me a design for one by email, which my sister and I reviewed and adjusted to make it appropriate for our family. In considering our choices, I spoke with my sister several times on the phone.

"The star's a little big," I said to her in our first conversation. "'Cahn' looks too big to me too. Maybe we can make them each smaller and then the names a little taller. What do you think?" I asked her. For I had felt that, in the monument company's design, the Jewish star and the family name overwhelmed the individuals. My sister agreed.

Later I called my sister to ask, "Should Minnie be 'Cahn Wasserman' or 'Wasserman, Sister'? How will people know her relation to us—that she was father's sister, not our sister?"

"They'll know by the dates," Kathe said, reassuring me.

"It doesn't really say who Danny was," I brought up. "'Son' isn't much." I was concerned that Danny, who died at age thirty-two and was our special younger brother, was not adequately represented. But more than that, I was concerned about our mother. "It doesn't say what mother did," I told my sister, feeling pained by the omission. "It says that father was a writer, but we don't say what mother did for work. Can we add 'teacher'?"

"She wasn't a teacher," my sister said gently. "She was a school psychologist."

"'School psychologist' would be too long," we both agreed, and, in my mind, I was still thinking teacher, remembering my mother from when I was very young when she worked as a nursery school teacher and was proud of her progressive approach. I also always felt my mother was a teacher in relation to me. Instructive in her style, she had taught me a lot about life.

"Father identified as a writer," my sister explained. "Mother identified as a woman no matter what she did. Those other things weren't central to her identity in the way 'writer' was for father. And 'teacher' just is not correct."

"Okay," I said, feeling amazed at my sister's insight and that she knew my mother far better than I did.

I then asked her, "Hannah thinks it's very patriarchal to have father's last name on top and his inscription coming first. Do you think so too?"

"I don't," Kathe said thoughtfully. "You could see it that way, but most people will see it as a family name. They will think, here is a family."

"Can we get rid of the family name, 'Cahn,'" I asked one of the monument company brothers when I next spoke with him. "Or is that usually what's done?"

"It's what is done," he said.

"Then leave it," I said, "but make it a bit smaller."

The star was made smaller, the "Cahn" made smaller, and the letters for the individuals were made slightly taller, though all of these changes were subtle.

I had not thought much before about the significance of calling a gravestone a monument, nor felt the importance of what might be inscribed on a stone's front. I had not thought of myself as a person who would be interested in cemeteries, yet now I was. When the new gravestone was set in place, I wrote to my mother's brother, who lived nearby, to tell him it was there, because I thought he would like to go visit it. I sent him a picture that showed the design of the stone with the inscriptions. I hoped he would approve of our choices and that he would feel the gravestone did my mother justice. He wrote back: "The design is perfect and the concept was wonderful. I will certainly stop by soon."

Before, I had visited my mother in the nursing center of her residence. Before that, I had always visited her at her home. Now it would be the cemetery.

It is my mother's birthday today, March 29. She would have been eighty-nine. Although she died over a year ago, her death feels quite recent to me. I am still wearing her bracelet. It rarely leaves my right wrist, and when it does, I put it in my left pants pocket, because I don't want to be without it. I am afraid that if the bracelet is not with me, I will have bad luck. At the same time, I fear that wearing it will bring me bad luck, that it will bring me my mother's luck, which is bad because she died—needlessly, I still feel. I think that the medical profession should have been able to save her, to avoid the drugs that may have damaged her lungs and to rid her body of the extra fluids that accumulated. But they could not. It saddens me and I miss her.

I have been wearing my mother's bracelet for five months now. The longer I wear it, the more accepting of her I become, not of her death, but of her life—how she lived, who she was. My mother is a hard woman for me to accept, because I have tried, in much of my life, not to be like her. With her bracelet, I sense that I am carrying this important piece of her around with me very obviously. I feel that I am her in some way, and that I owe that to her—to remember, to carry on who she was. I have wanted so often not to do that—not to be erratic, aggressive, harsh, demanding, commanding, brusque in my movements, dismissing of others, sharp, critical of so much around me, someone for whom things are not quite right. I have wanted to be a gentler person, more like my father perhaps, more content and more settled within myself and desiring to avoid conflict with others.

My mother did have many good qualities. She was smart—she knew the names of all the flowers, she remembered any detail she had ever heard. She was generous. She gave presents. She always had plenty of food for guests. A neighbor once gave her the shirt off his back and she thought that was how people should be. She was sentimental and caring. She was also easily hurt, but she did not let that get her down. She was strong in the face of adversity. However, my mother's good qualities are not the ones her bracelet confronts me with, but, rather, her more difficult ways, the qualities I do not wear as easily.

On Thanksgiving day this past year, for example, I got into an argument with several people, or at least a disagreement, and I ended up giving them a lecture on why I thought I was right, holding forth as my mother might—telling everybody off implicitly in my mind, setting the record straight, "being there" in my mother's way— superior-sounding, opinionated, brooking no opposition. After I spoke at the table, there was quiet, everyone else shut up or related to me in a demurring manner. I felt bad about myself, that I had not spoken with the usual social niceties. I had been a little uncouth, out of the norm. I thought maybe it was because I had wine to drink on an empty stomach. But really, I think, it was because my mother had died just the year before, right after Thanksgiving, and someone at this Thanksgiving gathering was talking about her mother and no one seemed to care about mine. No one seemed to notice that I could not see the soup in the bowl in front of me so I put my hand accidentally right into it. I was sitting squeezed into a corner at the table so that my guide dog Teela would not scare the hostess's cat. I felt caught too much within myself.

It was on Thanksgiving weekend last year that my mother decided she wanted to die—that living the way she was living, with the fluid accumulating in her lungs and her body, and no hope for improvement, was not worth it. She told me this on the Wednesday before Thanksgiving. Hannah and I had taken both Teela and our pet dog, Esperanza, to the beach. I called my mother from there to share the ocean with her, because I knew she liked the shore, though she liked that other coast best, the eastern shore, where she grew up. I was standing on a cliff overlooking the Pacific Ocean near Half Moon Bay, with Teela a comforting presence beside me. The wind was raging, the surf was high and beautiful. I held the phone up so my mother could hear the ocean waves. She told me that they would not let her in the dining room of her residence because she needed her oxygen with her, and she sounded pained. I knew she had taken her oxygen there before. I wondered, had she acted badly the last time she was in the dining room, had trouble managing her food or her temper? She spoke to me of the oxygen, but I think she felt she was being shunned, ostracized by others. Possibly she needed more assistance than she was receiving. I knew my sister and her family had asked my mother to spend Thanksgiving with them on Cape Cod, but she had not felt up to the travel. She may have needed the medical attention of the nursing center.

"I can't hear it," she said to me when I held the phone up again for her to listen to the sounds of the ocean. "I want to die," she then said. "I am going to stop eating."

"Keep eating until I get there. I'll be back to visit you next week."

"It's not the same eating by myself," she said.

It was a sad day for my mother and an unbelievable and sad day for me. I did not want my mother to die. I did not think she should have to die just because they would not let her in the dining room. But life often hinges on less.

On Thanksgiving Day this year, with my feelings of loss not far beneath the surface, I became my mother and I told everyone off. I was secretly proud of myself even if publicly, socially, I felt embarrassed and that I had not acted as I wished. I had conflicted, stood out. In my mind, my mother always stood out. She was tall, superior in her attitude, definite in her style, emotionally appealing like an adolescent girl might be, I always felt—people responded to her. Yet she often commanded what she wanted rather than asking for it. She could suddenly speak out in a way full of anger or self-righteousness. I think she felt most herself when apart, when she conflicted with others, came up against what someone else might say or think. I had to learn, as an adult, not to conflict, that I would not lose myself if I agreed. I had to learn the social graces and manners that it seemed to me other people came by more naturally, the habits of fitting in. I still do try to stand out, but in a quieter way than my mother.

I am generalizing about her, and it feels odd and not right, because my mother is not here to correct me. What if I am wrong? The world will have a negative view of my mother. I think it is not terrible for me to have a critical view, because I am her daughter and I love her. However, I have never understood her well. My sister understands my mother far better than I do, perhaps because she takes after my father, having an even temperament that gives her acceptance and distance. I mostly make guesses about this mysterious, strident, outspoken woman, whose sentences seemed to come out of nowhere, this woman who lived with a deep sense of sadness yet spoke with a musical lilt in her voice that I have always loved, this often socially difficult woman who was my mother.

I think that my mother had profound emotional disturbances within her that were beyond her control. These were covered thinly with the social graces she had learned from her mother and with her aspirations to be well thought of, to achieve status and security, and to contribute to the progressive causes in which she believed. I think she frequently felt at risk internally or endangered, and then she struck out at the outside world—verbally or by going into action—in order to protect herself, to feel competent and in control. I think she did not get along smoothly with people because she wasn't able to, not because she had a real choice. She was different and others had to give her some slack. You couldn't have quite normal expectations of her. You had to take her as she was. You could argue with her, but you should expect not to win.

I am going to wear her bracelet today when I teach my first class of the spring quarter, although I fear it will bring me bad luck—that when I open my mouth to speak, my mother's voice will come out and I will say something awful. I'll sound too superior, too definite, too confused; I'll seem harsh and uncaring even when I do care. I have had these same fears in anticipating two recent book talks I have given since beginning to wear my mother's bracelet. These were talks about my book, *Traveling Blind*. In preparing for each, as I looked down at the Navajo bracelet shining on my wrist, I saw my mother standing before people at a memorial for my father after he died. She was up on a stage, and, as she spoke, the right emotion was in her voice, and her tone conveyed authority, but her sentences did not connect. It was understandable after a death, but also, this was my mother. I fear I will speak in a similar manner—be both too confident and too confused.

As I dressed for my book talks, both times, I considered removing my mother's bracelet and changing it to one of mine—silver Navajo, of course, but a bracelet not cursed or blessed by the memory of my mother and the specter of her unpredictable outbursts. I stood at my desk, where I keep jewelry in my top drawer, slipped my mother's bracelet off my wrist and replaced it with my own—a bracelet with a more modern design and a central turquoise stone. I lay my mother's bracelet down on the desk, saw it looking abandoned and simple. Then I took my bracelet off and slipped my mother's back onto my wrist. I decided I wanted not to act in fear, but, instead, to go into the fray with this reminder, this part of myself, the different part that does not quite fit. I wanted to be strong enough to be myself even when, in part, my mother.

At the second book talk, held at a major civic club, although I had practiced my talk beforehand, I was particularly self-conscious and worried about what I would say. Would my sentences each have an end? Would I speak personally enough and yet generally enough? Would I get lost in some inner space of meaning? Would I answer the questions with proper respect? As I stood before the audience that evening with Teela lying at my feet, a bit of makeup on, wearing my better clothes and my mother's silver Navajo bracelet, I spoke from within myself and felt my words were my own. I did well. In the end, the people present applauded appreciatively, and I thought that my mother would have been proud of me. No matter what I said, it was that I said it, that people liked me, that I stood up before people and was accomplished and admired, and my mother was there with me. She was on my wrist beaming, glowing silver with feathers. She was right there beside me, not understanding me, as I do not understand her, but proud of me nonetheless. And I was proud because I had done it while wearing her bracelet and despite my fears that I would misstep, speak in some awkward way. I did okay and my mother was present with me, though perhaps not my real mother, but a benevolent and approving one.

I HAVE, ALL MY LIFE, studied my mother, trying to figure her out. I have worried about her, watching out for her. My sister and I often have treated my mother as if she was an egg with a hard shell that might crumble at any moment, causing the soft inner portion to flow out. We have sought to keep Humpty Dumpty intact, sitting high on her brick wall. Luckily for all of us, my mother kept her perch almost all the time. And we, or at least I, looked up from below, admiring her and seeking to do as she wished.

"Take this here." "Do this or that," my mother would say, and I would do it when I was not arguing with her—carry the dishes from the kitchen to a box in her living room to pack them up to give away—because these were dishes she no longer used, and she did not want anything extra complicating her life. "Just do it," my sister said to me that last time when I was visiting my mother back East before she went into the nursing center—on that visit when we thought she was fine. She was short of breath, but she thought she simply had to do more exercises to build up her stamina and that then her breathing would become normal. That was my mother—feeling the world was in her control, and, if it was not, she would make it so.

On my mother's birthday last week, her brother, Herbert, who is ninety-four, wrote to me:

Today was my beautiful sister's birthday, and I find myself the only one who can remember the day that lovely newborn came home from the hospital in 1922. Hospital births were somewhat new in those days. I was born at home on Kensington Street in New Haven in World War One time during food and fuel rationing and a deadly flu epidemic. Rhoda came home to a new house and to much love in a much more peaceful time. She was a beauty all of her life. It is sad that life was not more beautiful for her. I miss her badly.

My sister wrote back to Herbert saying that my mother was in her life daily and mentioning that I was wearing one of my mother's silver bracelets. I mentioned that, too, when I wrote to him, though I doubt he could have understood the significance.

My mother's bracelet sits comfortably on my right wrist. On my right ring finger, near it, is a silver Navajo ring of sandcast design with curved intertwined double-heart shapes that Hannah gave to me several years ago to match one that my aunt Minnie gave her back when she first met her, marking Hannah's acceptance into our family. This was a family not prepared for lesbianism, and Minnie did what my mother could not do outright.

My sandcast ring, which dates from the 1960s, is different in style than my mother's hammered silver bracelet, but the two go together, shining nicely. Both pieces are substantial in size and weight. I sometimes wonder how I can wear so much metal and not feel weighed down by it. But it feels fine. On my left ring finger, I wear a silver ring of Hopi overlay design given to me by Hannah on one of our first trips to New Mexico, marking something special between us. I also wear silver earrings.

My mother liked silver. She liked to put it on prominently and to take care with how she dressed so that she would look dignified and tasteful, with colors that complemented her skin tones. She especially liked blue, which a color advisor once told her was a good color on her. When I wear her bracelet with a light blue shirt, I feel I am almost her. For when I was growing up, she used to wear a light blue shirtwaist dress with the Navajo bracelet and a matching pin that my sister now has. The light blue of the dress brought out the gleam of the silver bracelet and made it look soft and appealing. I think this bracelet is best worn with blue.

When I wear it, I am constantly aware of where it is on my arm. Throughout the day, I check on it, as I once checked on my mother. I don't want to lose the bracelet or damage it. I don't want it to slip off my wrist accidentally if the opening gets turned around. I want to avoid its getting caught on something like a car door handle that might pull it off. I have learned to move my right arm and hand carefully to protect the bracelet from catching or scratching on surfaces like counters and walls or a flower pot I may be carrying. When I am out on the street walking with Teela, I check on the bracelet frequently to make sure it is still there, safely inside my jacket sleeve, and I rearrange it if needed. When I do dishes or manual work in the yard, I remove the bracelet and place it in my pocket, then check on it at intervals to make sure it is safe. When I finish my task, I put it back on. I don't want to keep it hidden for long. I don't want to be ashamed of my mother. I want to feel proud of her, that she is safe with me. I want not to fear her legacy.

For a small thing, this bracelet occupies a good deal of my attention. I would have thought I might begrudge it that attention, for I have always feared that if I paid too much attention to my mother, it would ruin my life. My mother, with her habits of aggressiveness toward me, has made it hard for me in an internal way, but I don't think I am ruined. She has also given me an invisible strength, and I would not want to be other than I am, even with my self-doubts.

Last year, two months after my mother died, I went back East to visit my sister to go through some of my mother's things that Kathe had taken back home with her to Delaware. On that visit, I sat on the couch in my sister's living room—with Teela lying peacefully at my feet—surrounded by furniture that had once been my mother's. In front of me was a small, round coffee table of my mother's—a modest maple wood table with decoratively carved legs that my sister and I have always liked and associated with my mother, for it reflects her simple yet classic taste. On a side table next to me was a brass lamp with a cloisonné inlay design that my mother seemed always to have had as well. My sister, sitting on a chair across from me, soon took out and placed on the round table several small silk bags and two boxes containing my mother's jewelry. This was not a great deal of jewelry, but a small collection of treasured pieces that my mother often wore. My sister and I began going through the jewelry, trying to identify the pieces.

"This was Grandma Gert's," my sister said, holding up a blue necklace that had belonged to my mother's mother and that my mother had liked. "I wonder what it's made of," Kathe said. "What is the blue stone, and is the metal gold?" I was aware that we did not now have my mother around to ask her. She would certainly know, and she would be able to tell us exactly when and where the necklace was made, what kind of trend in jewelry design it reflected, and who gave it to whom and when. She would be able to identify all the pieces and to tell us the story that went with each. And neither my sister nor I had inherited her particular fine mind for such detail.

A yellow silk pouch that my sister had placed on the table held most of my mother's silver jewelry. Kathe zipped it open, reached in, and handed me a pair of silver earrings with a curved, solid shape that my mother used to wear, often with the Navajo bracelet. "Go try them on," Kathe urged. I carried the earrings into the bathroom to look at them on myself in the mirror. They were snap-ons and possibly too heavy for me, but I liked them. They seemed to me so like my mother. I asked my sister to hold onto them for me and not give them away. I thought maybe I would take them someday and have them made over for my pierced ears. But taking them now felt too soon, as if it would mean that my mother had truly died.

By the time of my visit in February, my sister had already gone through my mother's jewelry with her three daughters. She did that very soon after my mother died, wanting each of her daughters to pick some things to remember their grandmother by. So some pieces of my mother's jewelry were missing from the collection. One was the silver Navajo bracelet. My sister's oldest daughter had taken it. It took me a while to ask for it, for I did not want any squabbles or hard feelings over material things to follow upon my mother's death. I did not want to take from my niece something she wanted for herself. But I wished to see the bracelet again, to try it on. When I asked my sister, she said the jewelry had been mainly pretty things for her daughter that caught her eye and that she would be pleased to send it to me. It took some time, but her daughter Rachel eventually gave the bracelet to my sister, who sent it to me in a large cardboard box full of packaged snack foods so that no one would know the precious contents. When I received the bracelet this past fall, I was so happy.

Two months later, when Hannah, Teela, and I were on our annual trip to New Mexico, we stopped into a trading post in a small mountain town. The trader, seeing my mother's bracelet on my wrist, quickly took out a rack of silver Navajo bracelets of a similar style to show me. "They're not as big," he said, handing two of them across the counter. They were lighter and simpler than mine. None of them had stamped feathers. They felt to me more recent and cheaper. I was amazed that they had a price attached to them, since I have always felt that my mother's bracelet is priceless. I was also dismayed that the price for them was modest. My mother's bracelet could not be worth that little, I thought, but I dared not ask.

I offered to take my mother's bracelet off and hand it to the trader so he could take a closer look at it. "I don't need to see it," he said. "I've seen lots of them." I felt shocked and hurt. How could he have seen my mother's Navajo bracelet before? It wasn't like any other. It had stamped feathers on it. It even had "whirling logs"— old-fashioned pre-World War II swastika-like symbols that were on the tips, although, fortunately, they had been worn off by use so that they were almost indiscernible, but I had looked them up. My mother's bracelet was heavy. It had significant weight to it. I was offended by the trader's indifference. At the same time, I knew that he had been in business for close to forty years so, of course, he had seen "old pawn" 1930s carinated, silver Navajo bracelets before, and his comment could be taken as indicating the authenticity of my mother's bracelet, confirming its value.

I am looking forward to my next visit with my sister when I will sit again in her living room going through my mother's things. I will perhaps take a few more pieces of my mother's jewelry. Kathe has said that her daughters can bring back the jewelry they took so that I can visit it. It's funny how jewelry can recall a person, especially pieces worn over many years. Perhaps I will also take the turquoise and coral Indian necklace I once gave my mother that, last time, we found she still had. It matches one I have. Maybe Hannah will wear it. It reminds me of giving my mother things when I lived in the Southwest. It was hard for me to see that necklace last time. My mother was gone, yet this piece of jewelry I had given her was still there, waiting to be given back.

For a long time after my mother died, my sister wore a ring of my mother's—made of diamonds and sapphires in a platinum band that had once been my grandmother's. My sister put the ring on right after my mother died. She also began to wear, on special occasions, an elegant silver bracelet of my mother's showing a bird eating fruit from a tree. That bracelet is larger than mine with a curved shape and a matching pin. Though not Navajo, it is striking and very much my mother. Kathe had an extra safety clasp made for it so she would not lose it from her wrist. When I started wearing my mother's Navajo bracelet, my sister told me about her wearing my mother's ring right after she died, and how, at some point, she stopped wearing it. I wondered if I would someday no longer wear my mother's Navajo bracelet. I did not want to imagine that, as if I would suddenly lose her again were I to remove it—lose my way of keeping her alive. Her bracelet has become a kind of monument for me, not big like a gravestone, but large in my mind—a woman's monument, a telling, intimate reminder.

Another such reminder that I noticed after coming home from my sister's was that often in my daily life when I pass a mirror, particularly the mirror in our bedroom—which is small and older and has a soft reflective quality, set in a wooden picture frame that my father once found at a flea market—when I pass this mirror and turn to look at my face, I will catch a glimpse of a certain cast of my eyes and I will see my mother. I used to see my father when I looked in mirrors. Now it is my mother. My eyesight is poor, so I see with much blurriness, but I can pick up the suggestion, the similarity. When I look at photos of myself magnified on my computer screen, I will sometimes also see my mother there. But it's in the mirror, in that quick glance to the side at that cast of my eyes that I suddenly find her staring back. Sometimes I look in the mirror just to see her.

My mother's silver Navajo bracelet sits on my wrist. It dates from the 1930s and has distinguishing stamped feathers. It was given to my mother by her husband's sister's mother-in-law and given to me by my sister's oldest daughter—on loan to all of us from history and from an unknown Indian silversmith long ago. I wrap myself in it, keep company with it, and look forward to when I will next visit my mother's memory in my sister's house. Kathe and I will open the pouches, take out the jewelry, and talk of old times. Handling the pieces, we will remember our father and our brother as well as our mother. I will finger the silver earrings my mother wore. I'll look at the pin that goes with the Navajo bracelet, made with a similar stamped design, and debate whether to take it, or whether to leave it in the collection, because maybe my sister will wear it more than I.

I will sit with my sister and think of my mother and be sad and, at the same time, proud that I had this difficult, strong, Jewish mother, this volatile, decorative personal heritage. I think my mother would be glad that I am wearing her bracelet—glad and pleased. She would also, while sitting at my sister's kitchen table, turn to me and say, "It's not the only kind of jewelry, you know, Suz. There are other kinds. You might branch out." That was my mother, knowledgeable, ever vigilant, always trying to improve me.

I am going to wear her bracelet, take care of it, and make sure it is safe, this flash of silver on my wrist. And as I do so, I will wrestle with my recurring fears about those parts of myself that remind me of my mother and that I often try to push away, concerned they will make me feel embarrassed, awkward, or unsafe. Perhaps one function of her bracelet is to help me to externalize—to hold outside myself a sense of inner threat, enabling me to keep my mother with me yet at arm's length—glowing, poised, to be cherished and admired, but never allowed to undermine me, as my mother once did. Her bracelet can be a reminder for me that I should seek the good, the glowing, the special, and turn away from the fears. I think my mother would have wished that.

November 2010–April 2011

TEN

$\leftlozenge\cdot\leftlozenge\cdot\blacklozenge\cdot\lozenge\cdot\rightlozenge$

Visiting Her Memory

As I walked toward the apartment building where Marion lived, I noticed that the drapes around her windows were closed—those windows that had always been open, the light coming through. Marion did not come to the front lobby to greet me as usual, so I went down the hall and knocked on her door. Occasionally before, she had fallen asleep late in the afternoon and I woke her when I knocked. I thought perhaps that had happened again. When no one came after repeated knocks, I went out to the front office of the residence where a manager told me, flat out, that she had died two days before. A day afterward, her cat had died. I was stunned. I had not expected this and, at the same time, I believed it all too easily, as if, of course, she had died. But there was never an "of course." I knew that Marion had been a smoker, and that, for several years, she had been on oxygen from chain smoking most of her life. But nothing had indicated to me that she was close to death. Marion was very alive for me, as she always had been. And yet she wasn't. It was chilling.

As I walked home, I was unsure how I would manage with the news, with this change in my life, this loss. In a way, it was time, I thought. Perhaps I had outgrown the relationship. Recently, I had had difficulty talking to Marion. I was less trusting of what she would tell me or that she could help me. We had trouble relating to each other. These difficulties made me very sad. And now she was gone. Like that. No warning. No one really to talk to about it. Our relationship had been so unusual, so involving, not like any other I had known. Not only did I need Marion in a deep way, but she had needed me. And in the end, I think she needed me more than I did her, or more than I could allow.

A week later, there was a memorial service for her in the meeting room in her residence, attended by people from the building and friends. I brought flowers and wine and spoke briefly about what Marion had meant to me. I was the only one there who was a client of hers, as far as I know. I think I was the only psychotherapy client she had at that time, for she had long since left the hospital clinic where I first met her and had been working out of her home in a semi-retired fashion. I think she saw other people at first when she left the clinic, but it was never something we discussed.

At the ceremony, after people had spoken of their memories of Marion, I stepped over to a side table to get refreshments. I laid my white cane against a back wall and turned to James, her best friend, a gay man, and soon began telling him that I was going to get a guide dog. I had filled out the application from Guide Dogs for the Blind just two weeks before—four days, in fact, before Marion died. I had been thinking about doing this for some time and particularly on my way over this afternoon—that I would get a Golden Retriever guide and no longer have to walk alone.

On my walk home after the ceremony, I thought, almost aloud to myself, "I will get a golden dog," remembering that Marion had golden blond hair, though it was graying. "I will replace her with a dog," I thought. "I will keep the dog with me now that she is gone." I only regretted that Marion would not be around to meet my new friend. This dog was going to carry her spirit. She would be abiding. She would be always with me, enabling me to feel the security, the sense of being less alone that I had felt with Marion. And, indeed, when Teela arrived six months later, she was soon always by my side, my companion, my tall, very solid accompanying presence.

The last time I spoke with Marion before she died, she said to me, "I don't want you to feel abandoned by me." "I don't feel abandoned," I replied, not knowing fully what she meant. I think she may have had an idea of the gravity of her physical condition of which I was unaware. I had not seen her for over a week because she needed time to recover from an injury to her knee after a fall. But I expected to see her the following Thursday. I did not think I had to call to check before our appointment. So I turned up that Thursday. The drapes were closed, and she was gone.

Who was Marion? What did she represent for me? She was my psychotherapist for eighteen years. She stirred my feelings about lesbianism and being different, my needs for someone outside myself, my needs to bring another person close, to have the intimacy that is often hard for me to achieve. Perhaps she represented the unattainable, yet I had a relationship with her of unparalleled presence in my life.

I first met Marion when she substituted for my regular psychotherapist in a hospital mental health clinic. She had called to ask why I was not seeing someone while my therapist was away. Her voice on the phone was definite and commanding. "What's going on?" she asked. "I wanted to see someone twice a week," I said. "I'll look into it." She soon called me back. "I'll see you Monday and Thursday." When I met her, I was surprised by how small her office was—a cubicle with a desk and two chairs, the desk piled high with file folders and books. Marion sat at the desk turned sideways toward me, so close that our knees almost touched. The closeness felt reassuring, enabling me to feel more connected with her, more willing to trust.

Marion was a small woman, but, from the start, she seemed large to me—self-assured, in charge, someone to be reckoned with. She was the chief of psychiatric social work in the clinic. Older than me by fourteen years, she wore slacks and a man-tailored shirt, open at the neck. Her sporty style of dress made me wonder if she was perhaps a wealthy woman who lived in the forested section of the city and either rode horses in her spare time or had cultivated a slightly upper-class style. Only later would I find that she was just the opposite of wealthy—a daughter of artists, a musician in her basic nature and talents who played the viola and had perfect pitch. She was a woman of modest means, though repeatedly over the time that the clinic was running she had offered to have her salary cut so that they would not have to lose other psychotherapeutic staff. She was also a lesbian, not at all a member of the heterosexual social world as I had first supposed. It took me a while to ask, but when I did, as if throwing caution to the winds, she told me she was indeed a "gay lady." She had short, sandy-blond hair in small curls.

As I sat with her in those first few weeks, I kept trying to figure her out. She seemed a mystery—this woman so close to me, yet so different—reaching out to me with her deep, resonant voice, demanding that I let her take care of me, that I let her oversee me and check things out. Right away, she wanted me to keep a log of my sleep—how many hours I slept each night, what it was like. I found it odd and unnecessary. I did not want anyone telling me to keep a log, and I did not do it for more than a week. It was my first exposure to the fact that Marion liked to assign numbers to things. "Where is that feeling on a scale of 1–10?" she would ask, leaving me to wonder and to question the desirability of the request, because I did not want my feelings made into a number. Like many things Marion tried to do with me at first, I challenged her and pushed it away, thinking I was educating her about how something ought to be done. One of the challenges I made to her concerned her desire to address me as "Miss Krieger." Since she was Miss Gerard, I would be Miss Krieger—possibly to equalize the relationship, possibly because that is what she had always done, or that was the custom where she came from. She was trained in the psychoanalytic tradition and there was a formality to it, though she had developed her own more interactive style. She had her degree as a psychiatric social worker from back East, had worked at hospitals with seriously mentally ill patients and at Yale University with "the docs," as she called physicians. I felt that therapy in the psychoanalytic tradition could unearth disturbing things within a person and that the transference dynamic could be disturbing as well, both prospects that scared me. Yet here I was entering into such a relationship.

When I told Marion that I did not want to be called "Miss Krieger," we went back and forth about it for some time. I must have argued, trying to persuade her. For I saw her as being a bit behind the times. I would educate her and bring her up to date. My psychotherapy experiences before had been more relaxed in terms of formal rules. I soon had her calling me "Susan" and I called her "Marion." At the time, I did not take her willingness to do this as a sign of her desire to please me, to be close to me, to have our relationship work, but I do think it was. Marion referred to the people whom she saw as "patients" and would continue to do so even when she was no longer working in a medical clinic but out of her home. I was used to being called a "client" and I tried to convince her to change that too, but she never did. I told her that I did not want to probe too deeply into my past, for I wanted to stay more in the present, to which she agreed.

From the start, Marion was willing to read my writing. The therapist I had seen before had not been willing to do that, so I was extremely grateful. I had recently completed a novel and Marion took it from me hungrily. When she finished it, she wrote me several pages of longhand notes about her responses to my main character, "Jenny," who represented me. She was very positive about Jenny, and about me. I have her notes about the novel in a file folder in my closet. I do not reread them because that would be too painful—causing me to wonder about my past and what it means and to feel the loss of the relationship between us. But I know the notes are there, and they convey the essence of Marion's positive attitude toward me—her desire to help and heal me, to be there for me, not to abandon me, and to have me present in her life as well. There is one sentence in the notes where Marion writes that she finds Jenny "loveable." At the time, that meant so much to me, and it's what means the most still.

After several months, I asked Marion if she would become my regular therapist. I had only recently come to the clinic when the long-term therapist I had previously seen elsewhere had to withdraw from practice due to illness. At the clinic, the first therapist I saw was helpful, but she did not relate with the depth that Marion did, which I needed. During the first year I met with Marion, my former long-term therapist died of her illness. My younger brother also died, a probable suicide. As I crossed the street on my way to the clinic the rainy afternoon my brother died, I almost ran, so eager was I to see Marion.

Over the years that I shared my life with her, other losses in my surroundings were less tangible than those initial deaths, but I continued to experience tumultuous emotions. I did not want to burden my relationship with my partner Hannah with all my internal distresses. The therapy, I felt, would be the place where I would work these out. At the start of this process, I sometimes lashed out at objects at home and broke them—the vacuum cleaner, a coffee mug or plate—trying to display my grief, frustration, or helplessness, my sense of things gone wrong, of having my needs unmet. In time, I no longer broke things. Maybe the change would have occurred without my seeing Marion, but I know that the two did correspond.

The personal history that brought me to Marion, and indeed to see psychotherapists for most of my adult life, is related, I think, to my early relationship with my mother, who—wonderful and smart and talented as she was—also had emotional disturbances deep within her that she passed on to me. Her ways of relating to me were often implicitly aggressive or distancing. As a result, I have long had to deal with forces within myself that I feel are attacking or abandoning me. These intensely self-critical inner voices make me doubt my own safety. Over time, I have had to learn how to talk back to the potentially destructive voices to settle inner emotional distress and to maintain a positive sense of myself. Because I have a challenging internal life, psychotherapy has been extremely helpful in enabling me to feel less alone with the emotional work I must do. It provides a sense that someone else is there with me, grounding me and affirming my worth and capabilities.

Because my mother's behaviors were erratic, it was hard for me to know when her striking out would occur—whether she was someone I could turn to or simply a hostile or abandoning force. What Marion offered me from the start in terms of simple constancy soon spoke to my needs. She seemed to understand my difficulties in trusting both others and myself and in feeling safe in the world, and she responded in the way she structured our sessions and our time together. Her approach was extraordinarily generous and was, I think, in keeping with the tradition she came from, which emphasized "doing what was needed" in response to a patient.

I saw Marion twice a week at first, then three times a week, on a sliding scale fee basis. Marion spoke with me on the phone one day of each weekend, usually Saturday morning at ten—to help me maintain a sense of connection with her. She also spoke with me on the phone sometimes during the week if I was upset. I would call her to try to fix what was wrong, to feel she was there for me and could help me. That sense of her "thereness" was at the heart of my therapy. The main form it took over all those years was a process of my reaching out to Marion to feel a connection with her, to be reassured by her constancy, and then of her responding, reaching back.

Very vivid in my mind are those times when Hannah and I were traveling in New Mexico and I would call Marion from afar. I have visions of myself, to this day, standing out in a phone booth in the middle of nowhere before starting onto a dirt road leading into the mountains, in a small town on a wood deck outside a country store, or in an isolated gas station early Saturday morning, trying to feel a connection with her. I would tell her where I was and how I was doing, seeking in her voice the reassurance I needed—that she cared about me, that I was not alone in confronting my inner churnings. I used to plan the stops for my calls carefully, scouting out the phone booths in advance, making sure the phones in them worked, then waiting there for the time of my appointment. One morning as I stood in Albuquerque in a dusty parking lot in front of a restaurant, soon after I picked up the phone, Marion told me, "I don't want to hear that you are having trouble. I want you to tell me that you are having a good time. That's what your therapist needs to know." From then on, I did as she requested. Though I did ask her, "Can I tell you first that I am having a good time, then something about the troubles?" "Of course."

Once when she was away and I had to speak with another psychotherapist on call, that therapist said of Marion, "She really cares." That assessment of her stayed in my mind. I think it is true, and it helped me often over the years when I doubted that she would be there for me, or that her intentions or her understandings of me were what I wanted.

Marion initially recommended that I take medication. She generally liked to have medication prescribed for her patients, she said, because it evened things out or calmed them down and then the psychotherapy could proceed better. She had Thorazine prescribed for me at first for anxiety and then Xanax, but I soon felt that the medication was getting in the way—that it was a substitute for my relationship with Marion. I was turning to the pills for help rather than turning to her. I had to see a physician for the prescriptions, which introduced an outside person, further complicating our relationship. After those two early tries with medication, I did not take any more, nor have I ever wanted to since then. I felt better facing my problems more directly. Yet I greatly appreciated Marion's desire to put me on medication initially—because I felt it indicated that she was taking my emotional difficulties seriously.

In the first few years that I saw her, I was often easily upset, particularly upon leaving Marion and the warmth and protection she offered. One afternoon, I overturned two chairs in the clinic waiting room after our session, distressed about the parting, and about some unresolved difficulty between us. Marion was quite angry with me and asked that I bring flowers and apologize to the office staff. In retrospect, I am not proud of my behavior at that time. I was a grown woman and I upturned chairs in a clinic where children also came for supportive care, although the lobby was mostly empty that afternoon. Often after seeing Marion, I would sit on the steps leading down to the outside entrance to the building because I found it so hard to go back into the outside world. The first time Marion found me there, she stood close and gestured with her hand, bringing me back inside to talk it over in her office. She made me feel that my acting out could be superseded by my finding a way to talk with her. That was certainly the medication I needed.

Much of my distress during that initial period coincided with the clinic changing offices. When I first saw Marion, we sat very close together in her small office. When the clinic moved to new quarters a year later, her office was larger and our chairs farther apart. Marion seemed to think the distance between us was the same as before, or that it made no difference, but it made a difference to me. The extra space between us and all around us made me feel I was floating and that I was far away from Marion, and as if she had suddenly become a stranger. I felt that my heightened emotional difficulties stemmed from that added space. Of course, I knew there were deeper roots, but the acuteness of it seemed to have to do with the distance and with my feeling that I had lost an initial period of closeness, a fantasy, a dream in which we were as one. I don't think Marion believed me that the space in the office was a real problem, but I was glad when she moved to a small corner office down the hall where we sat closer. I felt more in touch with her there and more settled emotionally.

When the hospital closed the clinic for economic reasons, Marion began holding her practice in her home. For eleven of the eighteen years I saw her, I met with her in one personal residence and then a second, sitting across from her in the intimacy of her living room. I sat on the couch, Marion across from me on a chair, a coffee table between us or off to the side. I was driving at the time of her first home, but by the second, I was losing my eyesight enough so that I soon had to walk. Fortunately, Marion's second residence was close to where I live, close enough so that if I stood on top of the hill that rises at the corner near our house and took out my binoculars, I could make out her white apartment building in the not-too-far distance. I always swore to myself that if and when Marion died, or when I was no longer seeing her, I would move out of the city. There would be nothing keeping me there anymore. Yet she died and I still live in San Francisco. I hardly believe it possible that my life goes on here without her.

Not long after I began walking to Marion's, we had a session in which she began telling me how and where she thought I ought to cross streets on my route home. I balked. I argued with her. I did not want to be told how to cross a street. I wanted to be trusted, I told her. She then made clear that she was giving me this advice because she was worried about me. I had not thought that Marion would worry about my safety in her absence—my physical safety—although I had always wanted her to worry about my emotional safety. That day, as so often, I was trying to get Marion to respond as I wished, and she to get me to see it from her side, explaining and expressing her concern.

The core of our relationship—amidst all the moves and the comings and goings—was always that back and forth between us, as we sought to maintain the stability, reliability, in-touchness, of our relationship—the "holding" power of it, the feel of the bond. We tended our relationship as one might a growing plant, an injured animal, a young child missing a mother, seeking to heal, to make better, to relieve the pain I felt.

I always wanted Marion to give me a hug. At the end of every session, she would give me a handshake, as if that was her version of a hug. Her hands were broad; she had a firm grip—intentionally, I think—to convey to me all the emotional presence she felt and wished me to feel as well. Sometimes she referred to her hand as her "paw," a gruff way of referring to the affection that was not so gruff underneath. I wanted, from early on, to have her be less formal, more like other therapists I had known, who gave hugs easily. I wanted her not to be constantly announcing the presence of barriers, of a closeness where she would not go with me. So I asked her for a hug on many occasions. Instead, she gave me a handshake, ever more firmly each time, sometimes enclosing my hand in both of hers, as if saying with it, "I am here." Once on the phone, she said to me, "I am holding you as well as I can." I felt surprised. The image was so comforting. And it was not at a time when I had asked for that. But I think she knew what I needed. Over the years, I asked Marion for a hug at certain times more than others. Sometimes, she offered to consider it; at other times, she simply gave me a handshake. It was an issue with me—a repeated underlying longing—as if that hug that I did not get would solve everything and free me, in fact, from longing. Three times, Marion actually did give me a hug, and I can still feel her body against mine. Her breasts were soft yet firm; she was a solid, compact woman. I did not give her as full a hug in return. There was part of me, a big part—more than I knew and yet I knew it—that was not willing to be fully there.

I think Marion did not feel that a physical hug was necessary and she also did not think it was wise. The relationship between us was close enough not to have it confused by other things—sexual feelings, anything that would muddy the waters, that would detract from the therapy, blur the boundaries, get in the way of the work, the basic reliability of the bond. I remember one day I was sitting in her living room on the couch across from her—where I always sat in her second apartment—and the subject of the hug came up, and Marion said suddenly, "I wish we could ask Queen Solomina"—referring to the hug and wishing for wisdom from a female King Solomon as to whether it would be a good idea. I very much appreciated her wish, her request, and I understood, in that moment, the seriousness with which she guarded doing right by me. Still, though, I longed for the hug.

Once when I got a new puppy, Esperanza, Marion seemed to break all rules and came to visit at my house to meet her. She sat on a stool in the kitchen, picked up little black Esperanza and held her. "Bellissima Esperanza," she said. I was very moved that she came to visit. We sat in the living room and talked for a while as if in a therapy session. Then she came with me outside to my yard—as she had done once before to see my plants flowering in springtime—and together we watched Esperanza romp in the greenery. Marion was willing to do that extra—to come over to my house—more easily than giving me a hug, I felt. But it ran together. It all said how much she cared, how much she was willing to try new things, to demonstrate, to stretch her boundaries for me.

Toward the end of my seeing her, in the last couple of years, Marion sometimes fell asleep briefly during our sessions. She would suddenly drift off, then come to. I think she was not getting enough oxygen, even when she started receiving supplemental oxygen from a machine. She had been such a heavy smoker most of her life that, although she had recently stopped smoking, her lungs now had limited capacity. When she woke up after briefly falling asleep, she would act as if it made no difference, and then she would simply carry on with what we had been discussing. Sometimes, though, she would tell me about what she had dreamed. After a while, I felt as if it was normal for her to fall asleep occasionally, but I think it haunted me. It was unsettling deep down, causing me to feel afraid that I might be losing her and her abilities. When I first saw Marion, she still smoked, and she asked my permission to smoke during our sessions. I never minded. I always felt it was "Marion's smoke," so it was good. It made me feel surrounded by her, enveloped by her presence, and it made me feel I was where I wanted to be. But the smoking had effects, and, especially toward the end, I think I did not trust Marion enough because of that signal—that falling into sleep—as if it meant something was wrong, something was missing—and because of my tendency so easily not to trust. I began talking to Marion less and less in our sessions. This hurt her feelings. Once she cried because I seemed so withholding. She told me she felt rejected by me. Still, I seemed not to be able to do anything about it. I would sit there across from her and not talk much or deeply, simply stroke her cat in my lap as I searched for the words. The silences would be painful.

Eventually I cut back my number of therapy sessions per week from three to two. Marion did not think this was necessary or advisable, but it was what I did in an attempt to cut down the length of the silences—in the hope of making things better. I did not want to hurt Marion's feelings, and I have never gotten over a sense that I hurt her—by my withholding—and that I was a bad person for doing that. At the same time, I think I blamed her for my sense of loss—as if she should not have fallen asleep, should not have been who she was, should not have gotten older, or weaker, or less able to stir my deepest feelings, to make me trust her, rely on her, feel she was the most important person in my life other than Hannah. I never talked to Marion directly about how I felt when she fell asleep or had trouble breathing. Like her, I wished to ignore the difficulty, not let it detract from the therapy, not let it deter us, or change anything. I can see now that Marion may have so wanted not to abandon me, not to let me down, that she tried, even in those challenging circumstances, to come through—to be there for me. And I can see that I feared, and wished not to fear, that she was failing me.

While I was seeing Marion in her second home—walking there or taking the bus—I would often become afraid in the autumn when it began getting dark early. It was a rough corner on a busy street where I would have to wait for the bus on my way home, and I did not want anyone accosting me because I was a blind woman carrying a white cane, or attacking me while I was walking up the hill. As I left Marion's apartment on some of those late afternoons when it was dark and rainy, I so did not want to go out, but wished to stay longer in that warmth, that closeness. And yet I walked off, felt the cool air, the rain, disappeared into the crowd, into my own life.

I always felt that Marion was an unusual person with her own distinct views. She had her own mind, kept her own counsel. She played competitive bridge regularly at least twice a week and traveled to bridge tournaments. It was a serious avocation for her. When she was living with her long-term lesbian partner, they played and traveled together. I felt that doing something regularly that was abstract and involving was congruent with who she was. "If it wasn't bridge," she once told me, "it would have been the viola," which she used to play in string quartets.

Marion was from New York City. She had grown up on Staten Island before there was much settlement there and took the ferry daily to Manhattan to attend the High School of Music and Art. She was an only child, self-assured in a basic way, I felt, perhaps because she had a very devoted mother. Both her mother and her father were painters. Her father had been a founder of the *New Republic*, an early progressive magazine, and had died when she was young. Carrying on that heritage, she had left-wing political views, probably not characteristic of her bridge and social set, I thought. Our political views were something we had in common. "The wave of the future is backward," I once said to her and she liked that a lot.

Marion dressed differently than others, more individually, I felt, but like a lesbian of her generation. When I once told her I thought she was "butch," she seemed aghast and denied it. "I wear dresses," she said. "When?" "When I go to the opera." It was so like her. She did not believe in enacting male and female roles among women. It was something she had reacted to in her youth. Yet here she was, clearly not the conventional woman in style, not femme. Once she said to me when I was talking about a difficulty I was having with Hannah, "You know how to please your lady." The expression seemed to me "old gay" and made me want to do just that.

Marion had three cats when I first knew her. I had one cat and soon wanted to have three, and then did.

Marion's views on how to conduct therapy seemed to me different from those prevalent around her, more individually adaptive, less standardized. Our sessions, for instance, were an hour and a half each, rather than the usual fifty-minute hour, because Marion felt I needed the extra time. It took me fifteen minutes to feel I was there after I entered the room and sat down, and then, toward the end, I needed about fifteen minutes to prepare to leave. The coming and going was so important and so hard for me. Simply getting to Marion was often the main point. Similarly, on the phone, the beginnings and ends of our conversations mattered and were hard for me. They were always spaces I had to work out—how enter them, how leave them, how enter and leave Marion?

After Marion died, as I walked away from her apartment building the afternoon I heard the news, I thought about how she had been different. I knew I would be going down to the university the next week to begin my spring quarter's teaching. I wondered how I would be able to do it, having had this traumatic loss so recently.

I also feared, as I had sometimes before, that I was too much like Marion, too different in her way—too gruff, too old-fashioned, not conformist enough. I feared that Marion had been too unusual in her beliefs and style and that death had been her punishment for it. And I worried that just as I had withdrawn from her in certain ways, others would withdraw from me. I am not like her, I told myself that day, and yet I felt I was. I felt her presence all the more now that she was gone. I felt her vulnerability. I decided I would brave it, face the world, carrying her with me.

Once as we sat together in Marion's living room, she had taken off her eye glasses and looked at the bookshelves across the way. The titles were blurred. "I can't read them. Is that what it looks like for you?" she asked. Then she put her glasses back on. I think she was trying on what it might be like to be me, and I think I never fully enough grasped what it was like to be her. I kept wanting her to be me, or me to be her. I got the two intertwined. Now it's time to separate them, to pull us apart, but maybe not.

"Keep me with you in a positive way," Marion used to say to me. At first, it was simply, "Keep me with you"—her effort to help me maintain the connection when we were apart. I added "in a positive way," since I knew I tended to have the negative creep in, to doubt the goodness of her feelings for me. When my mother died—five years after Marion died—as I stood in a cemetery remembering my mother, searching for what to say to her, it came to me, "I will keep you with me in a positive way," I said, something so basic that I learned from Marion.

Marion used to read my writing regularly. After "Jenny's World," each book manuscript that I wrote I gave to her in advance. She liked my writing and compared it to music. I tried, each time I gave her a section or chapter, to get her to tell me how she felt upon reading it. She found that hard to do. What she really wanted to do, and I can see her doing this, was to raise her two right fingers in the air, pinch them together with her thumb, then spread them apart as if to blow a kiss. She was trying to convey the exquisiteness she felt. "It's music," she said. "How can I tell you about that?" Though repeatedly, she tried, because I asked. There was only one piece of writing I ever gave her that she did not like. That was a diary-like story I wrote while traveling in the Anza Borrego Desert, a narrative written at the time, with more about going from place to place and fewer layers of meaning than my usual writing, which is done when I am at home and in retrospect. She was right, I think. I never tried to write that way again. I knew Marion expected my writing to have deeper meanings, to sing, to flow, to be a symphony. It was music within me, and I was grateful it had felt that way to her as well, that she had put that into words. Often I did get her to put more words to how she felt upon reading. But it was the wordlessness, the general appreciation and her understanding of what my writing was about, what it conveyed, that mattered—and her willingness to welcome each piece of writing that I handed to her, to cradle it gently in her hands, and to look forward to reading it.

On the day I turned up for my appointment at Marion's apartment and found that she had died, I spoke with some people in the building who told me that she had continued to smoke even after she had gone on oxygen, which she often carried behind her in a canister on a small pull device. This came as a surprise to me. I thought she had completely stopped smoking, because that is what she led me to believe. She hid that from me. I think she did not want me to think less of her, or she may have wanted not to worry me. Once she told me there was a woman at bridge who had oxygen with her and smoked at the same time. I said I thought that was odd—never knowing it was possibly herself she was telling me about, as she waited to hear how I would respond. During the time I saw Marion, I know she made great efforts to stop smoking because of how it affected her breathing. But somehow she could not go through with it entirely. In the end, because of her long-term smoking, her heart failed.

In Marion's living room, there was a black, lacquered coffee table in front of me that she had made. She had also made the low black shelves on both sides of the room housing her record collection. On the side table to my left sat a tall lamp she had made from an old bronze fire extinguisher. It was magnificent. The day after I left the memorial service, I wondered what had become of her possessions. "I would have liked that lamp," I thought. It had lit the way for me, sat beside me, giving off a large, warm glow. I had to remind myself that it is not in a possession that I would remember Marion, but in what happened. And sometimes I do not want to remember—because I do not want to stir the loss, feel again that time before the end when I had such difficulty talking with her. When I think of how different I felt Marion was—old-fashioned, old-style dyke, having her own mind, playing bridge, smoking, putting herself out for me, seeing me in therapy in a very unconventional way by some standards—yet always retaining that clinical reserve to some extent, that distance—when I think of her constancy—I think often that she should not have cared so much. She shouldn't have stretched the limits—seen me three times a week, and those phone calls so often, and the hour and a half—and yet that is what I wanted. And she responded to me—was there for me. She was willing to be on the other end of my insecurities, not to have them scare her away, though sometimes she became irritated with me when something I did in relation to her seemed not right.

Our relationship was so unconventional. Marion gave to me so much more than people, especially therapists, usually do, and shared herself with me so generously. I needed and wanted all that she gave. The degree of connection I felt with her, the deep attachment, enabled me to feel less alone as I walked through the world. I felt as if surrounded by that glow from her lamp. Yet in her absence, I feel undeserving, and then the doubt creeps in. I wonder whether I gave her enough in return. I want her back to affirm, with her presence, the rightness of our pairing.

At Christmastime each year, Marion used to put up colored lights around her front apartment windows. I would see these lights framing the windows as I walked toward the building. She often left them up for two or three months afterward. "These are dark months of the year," she said. "Any extra light helps." During our sessions, she almost always had a front window open, letting in air. The drapes were rarely closed. When they were drawn that day I arrived and found her gone, it was such a contrast. I immediately felt something might be wrong, but that it was probably that she had fallen asleep.

Marion always offered me two tissues when I reached for one. "Take two," she would say as I leaned over toward the box on the table. To this day, when I reach for a tissue in my bathroom, I think, "Marion would have said, 'Take two,'" and then it is a challenge for me. Do I take two Kleenex and then I will have an extra that I surely will use since one is so flimsy and small and there is always a need for an extra tissue? Or do I take only one, trying to forget Marion, trying to separate myself, not to have her life, her death, her differentness so mark my own? Does Marion remind me of my mother, whom I often wished to push away, fearful of being her, of not fitting in, of losing myself to a larger presence, a more important presence than mine, fearing to fail her in what she wanted for me, or in what she wanted me to be? Perhaps it is that. Perhaps it was the nature of the tie—close but not too close.

I wish I could have talked to Marion more fully and deeply and truthfully in that last period before she died, and yet I cannot see myself doing so. I see myself as it actually was. I ring the front doorbell. Marion comes out to the lobby to meet me and we walk back to her apartment. Or I knock on the apartment door myself. When I greet Marion, she is always glad to see me, as if, finally, I have arrived. Then we sit down, settle in. She patiently waits as I begin to talk. Then she listens, trying to make sense of what I say, trying to respond in a way I won't reject, won't argue with her about.

"Why don't you slip your CV under the office door. Get down there first thing in the morning at 8 a.m.," she tells me. "They don't do that in academia when you apply for a job," I say. She seems miffed, or confused, or at least taken aback. We talk. I tell her about my walk over. I tell her about something I have been writing. I actually do not remember well the things I told Marion about, or her many thoughtful statements in response—the things she so carefully said—as if they were less important than my simply sitting there—with her, in her presence, feeling that she wanted me, always wanted me, to say more, to be with her, to give her material with which to help me. Once she apologized for not being a psychoanalyst. Maybe I would do better with that type of treatment, she suggested. But I never wanted that. I wanted exactly what she gave, I think, and even more—the hug, more closeness—so that in the end I would feel more free to talk—to explore those other realms. To give to Marion more. And in my fantasy, she would respond perfectly, always perfectly, never giving me advice that I didn't need, never doubting my ability to deal well with things.

Marion liked people. When she would hear about someone acting oddly or come across an angry motorist on the road, she would try to understand their anxieties, to psychoanalyze them. She was like my father in liking people, in feeling positive affection toward others generally, except for those few of whom she disapproved. She was steadfast, solid, sturdy. "I am in it for life," she said to me once in describing her relationship with her partner. When they broke up and I asked her about it, she told me, "I have not felt this much pain since my mother died."

After Marion died, I did not see another psychotherapist for a long time—until two and-a-half years later. I could not imagine it. It seemed too hard. How could I follow that depth of experience? And I needed to free myself. I also think I had a sense of Marion's strong presence within me. And I felt, how could someone else understand?

It was hard getting used to seeing the next psychotherapist, who did extremely well by me. But I was now in a traditional fifty-minute hour, with one session per week, paying full price, keeping up the formalities. I wasn't acting out in that way I had at first done with Marion. I wasn't pining for my new therapist when I was gone from her, constantly seeking to repair the connection. My deepest feelings and desires were not so close to the surface. They were more submerged, more under control. In our sessions, I spoke to fill the silences. I did not want another therapist to feel rejected by me because I did not talk enough. At the same time, I spoke of things more casually, more superficially. I spoke often about my guide dog. There was nothing wrong with that, but I knew I did not cry, or probe too deeply. I stopped being able to talk at one point, feeling at a loss for words, for an ability to connect, angry somehow. And then it affirmed how I had been with Marion. Perhaps the problem hadn't been Marion so much as me, I thought— my reluctance to disclose, my fears, my desires for closeness yet my tendency to pull away, to keep myself apart after an initial intimacy.

Marion used to say that I, and any patient of hers, was an "esteemed friend." I thought that expression quaint and old-fashioned, but it felt right. It suggested, at once, that closeness and the distance, the formality that found a hug too much. For something had to be beyond us.

I am back in Marion's living room with her, sitting on her couch. She is on a chair opposite me. The rug on the floor is a brown and black oriental. I do not yet have my guide dog Teela, so there is no golden hair on the rug. Yet sometimes I see myself there with Teela. Marion knew that I was planning to get a guide dog. I had asked her once how that would be for her. "If I got a dog, a Golden Retriever," I told her, "there will be hair on your rug." "I'll vacuum," she said.

One day two years after Marion died, I took a walk over to her apartment building, accompanied by my new guide dog, Teela. I had not been back since the memorial service. In front of the building, up near the sidewalk, was a small park. There was a broad plot of grass within it and a children's play area with sand and swings. I opened the gate from the street side and walked in, then sat down on a bench with Teela beside me. I looked across the adjacent parking lot toward the windows of the corner apartment that had been Marion's. The dark drapes were no longer there. Marion's blue vintage Volvo was not parked out in front. Or was it? I thought I saw it, though my vision is poor and that may have been wishful thinking on my part. I thought maybe someone in the building bought it. But Marion was not here, only my memories of her. I sat on the bench in the sun and thought about what I wanted to say to her. It was the perfect moment. No one was around. I could have said something out loud to her, some significant statement. I thought I would ask her advice. She might help me settle a current concern that was worrying me. But I have no idea now what that was. I was anxious, I know, but I did not say anything, as when I saw her, often I could not get words to come out—those words that would betray my needs. I simply thought of her and of the empty apartment. I thought, "What advice would she give me?" And in my mind, I heard her affirming whatever I was planning to do, saying it was all right, it was good. I should trust myself. I am not sure that Marion ever said those words to me, "trust yourself," but they were what came to mind. I could not get her to tell me more.

I stood and took a floppy Frisbee out of my backpack and walked over to the plot of grass and tossed it to Teela, who happily ran back and forth to retrieve it so I would throw it to her again and again. I was worried that someone would come out of the building and tell me that a dog could not play there, but no one came. I hoped, in part, that someone would come, because maybe they would remember me from all those years when I visited Marion. I imagined a resident looking out from an upper story window or peering out from the main glass front door of the lobby. I would have liked to reminisce, to talk with a person who had known Marion. But it was just Teela and me.

Once when I was seeing Marion, she mentioned that after dark a few times, a woman would come from somewhere in the neighborhood fairly late at night. She would come with her dog and a ball. She would throw the ball to the dog and the dog would chase it under the lights of the parking lot outside Marion's ground floor windows. Marion felt it was clear that the woman loved the dog and the dog loved the woman and that together they so enjoyed this play with the ball. Their feelings for each other were all expressed in the play. I saw, in my mind, the neighboring woman with her dog that evening, and I saw Teela in front of me, her golden hair glowing against the bright green of the grass in the sun as she retrieved her Frisbee. No one bothered us. They just let us play. In a way, Marion did that for me. She let me play. She let me be. She let me ask and ask again. She responded as best she could. She was constant. She was with me. She is with me still.

I see her looking out now from her corner window, reminding me that I had needed her and that she did not wish to leave, and that one day we would again sit together, talking back and forth, trying to work it out, consulting with Solomina. I miss her.

October 2012

ELEVEN

◆◆◆◆◆◆

Writing My Way through It

SOME YEARS AGO, I found online a discussion of my book *Social Science and the Self: Personal Essays on an Art Form* in which the reviewer said, "I want to be Susan Krieger." I was surprised and flattered. This seemed to me the highest compliment I could be given—that someone else felt my life was desirable enough to want it to be theirs. I had begun to write personally in that book, arguing for acknowledging the self of the researcher as a valuable resource within the social sciences, rather than viewing it as an undesirable contaminant. To illustrate my points, I discussed my writing of an earlier study, *The Mirror Dance: Identity in a Women's Community*, my feelings on interviewing others in social research, my graduate education, my sense of the value of psychotherapy, and the loss of my younger brother through suicide—reflecting on how these events had affected my work. I believe that my discussion of my own life experiences suggested they were often emotionally difficult, though that difficulty was repeatedly a source of growth for me, providing insights that helped me also to understand the lives of others.

When I read the reviewer's comment that she wished to be me, I was especially moved because it seemed that my difficulties in life had not scared her away, and her comment made me feel that, despite my doubts, I was an adventurous spirit. I saw myself riding off into the sunset—a cowgirl on a horse in a novel for teenaged girls, happy in the outdoors, setting out on new adventures, slaying enemies and dragons, taking readers with me. I was a smiling girl with curly hair. The horse was chestnut brown. We were together going off on an open-ended, exciting journey. I had an uplifted spirit and no questioning about the rightness of what we were doing. Further, I felt that the reviewer's phrase suggested a basic acceptance of me that I was unsure that I had for myself. Over the years, her comment has stayed with me, emerging occasionally, and coming to mind especially recently as I attempt to confront inner self-doubt.

My most troublesome doubt at the moment concerns my ability to write. I am afraid that I can no longer write, that the ability to connect words together, to put my thoughts into a string of associations that might be helpful or of interest to others, and meaningful to me, has slipped away, vanished, never again to be drawn upon. I am afraid that I will not be able to speak from my inner emotional depths, from those feelings just beneath the surface that I usually explore in my writing. I do so in order to be a candid person and to create something that might offer insights to others at the same time as this writing produces an inner self-enlightenment and freedom for me, an inner therapy and self-care. Yet I now fear that I will repeat myself, say something I have already said, that it will take me too long to write, that I will spend my time revising forever, that I will waste my time, expend it doing something that does not amount to much. I am afraid that I am getting older and losing all my abilities. That last is at the crux of this.

When I was initially losing my eyesight, I faced a similar writing dilemma. The words soon swam before me at the computer and I could not write my sentences because I could not see them. To write the first article I had due at that time, I asked for help from my partner Hannah, who read the words aloud to me when I needed it and went over each paragraph to check on my prose. She gave me feedback so that I could produce the article, which fortunately was short.

I was so overwhelmed by the newness of my extreme loss of vision that I was simply reeling with that, and not too worried about my writing. Though frustrating, I assumed the writing would become easier again, that I would learn new skills. Over time, I learned to write using large bold print on paper and my talking computer with its text-to-speech and magnifying programs. Even now, the time it takes to write and revise is challenging and often discouraging for me, but I feel that I can write despite my blindness. Still, I think that I underestimate the challenge of doing so. When writing takes me more time because I do not see well, when the computer work takes so many extra steps—and the voices of what I potentially might say swim in my mind, struggling to get out but feeling they have nowhere to go—I feel discouraged, but I don't want to admit it. I feel that I cannot write well, that the effort is perhaps not worth it.

In recent years, as my blindness has become worse, I find that my writing requires increased patience and persistence on my part as the letters become more cut up and invisible. There is less there on the page, more to compensate for. I have to learn how to write by listening to the flow of the words rather than by seeing them in print. I face new challenges. But I think that an additional obstacle frustrating my confidence is attitudes toward getting older that I have internalized. I somehow believe that as I get older, I will lose all my abilities, or at least the important ones, the mental ones so intimately connected with my ability to write. I believe that I am, at age sixty-six, suddenly "over the hill"—too old to write anything of significance, losing my grasp on the words, their meanings, losing my ability to draw from my inner depths to say anything useful, insightful, exciting, of interest to myself and others. I have swallowed wholesale the ageism around me. I have accepted that I am in decline, as if I have a death sentence and it starts now. I am about to die, so why try?

By comparison, when I began to lose my eyesight at age fifty-one, I did not as easily accept but, instead, recoiled from the negative attitudes that I felt all around me concerning blindness. I would not subscribe to them. I would not accept ideas people sometimes had that I was now more limited than before, worse off, or unfortunate. I would view my blindness as a difference and a welcome and positive difference at that. I would show how it helped me, made a new life for me. I gained a guide dog and with her a new sense of adventure.

But the specter of getting older does not seem as exciting. I do not view it with the same open possibilities. Probably because it is generally felt to be the one condition with a dead end. But I hope and think it must be more than that. I am not that different today than a few years ago. It's my outlook that is different. I want to counteract my internalization of the negatives surrounding getting older as I did the negatives surrounding my loss of eyesight. How can I do that? My way is to probe further beneath the surface of my emotions, where it seems to me that the sense of loss, incapacity, and life change that now disrupts my confidence in my ability to write is, in part, a product of my mother's death two years ago. And, more deeply, it reflects those churning internal forces I inherited or learned from her that all too easily are set loose within me.

I did not have these same feelings of inadequacy before my mother died. But several months afterward, when I sat down to write, thoughts swum in my mind and before me on the page, resonating in my inner ear as I heard what I was writing. I felt I could not organize my words well. What would my mother think? I felt afraid of alienating readers, rather than as if I was taking them with me on a new adventure that they would appreciate. I felt that I was no longer the teacher, leading the way with my writing, helping others to notice things I could see, helping others to value me, and me to value myself. I was the daughter trying to make peace with her distant mother. Immediately after her death, I wrote "On a Distant Hillside," discussing my last visit with my mother and the comfort I soon found on a trip to the New Mexico desert, where I sought to honor her memory and to recover from my loss.

But when subsequently I began writing "My Mother's Brace-let," my sense of my prose became increasingly confused. I was rearranging the words all the time, unsure of what would make my sentences better, doubting my ability to do so, to make the sentences clear, the flow of the whole work out. I was trying to sum up who my mother was with words, imagining her back. It was not a terrible experience, and it wasn't hard to get the words down in some form. But fixing them up, making the sentences and the whole into what it should be, was a challenge, and I wondered whether I could live up to it. I did finish "My Mother's Bracelet," and the writing seems to have conveyed my meaning and emotion—concerning how I felt making arrangements for my mother's gravestone, going through her jewelry after her death, then choosing to wear her treasured silver Navajo bracelet, which confronted me with settling turbulent parts of her also within me. That story worked out well in the end and readers have liked it. But it is the inner questioning, the self-doubt that pervaded my writing of it that bothers me, that stands out in my mind as I try to take on a new task—the next writing piece, the next chapter. I have far too much self-doubt getting in my way, too many self-critical inner voices telling me I cannot do it, saying my writing is wrong, criticizing my rhythm and my sentences.

My writing used to be a place where I relaxed and felt hap-piness, felt that if I just let the words flow, I would be creating something new and marvelous, or if not marvelous, interesting or insightful. I would look forward to showing my writing to others. Not that much seemed to stand in the way of the first draft—although there were many revisions—and the time when I could share it. But now so much seems to stand in the way. I think my moth-er's death knocked me out, shocked me, changed my world, made me feel what I had always felt in the face of my mother—possibly incompetent, questioning my own worth, viewing what was intrin-sic to me as foreign, to be hidden, not there. Her death has made me feel older, but I think it has made me feel far too old. It has made me feel I am my mother and that I am about to die. I have to find ways, instead, to be myself.

I know I have taken strength from my mother's positive qualities—her intelligence, her pride in life, her generosity toward others—but clearly I have also internalized her in deeply self-critical ways, carrying her with me in these ways in order not to lose her. I wear her within as surely as, on my wrist, I wear her bracelet. I think, too, that when my mother died, I lost a basic protection against negatives from the outside world and against my own self-critical inner voices. My mother was gone, and gone with her the presence that might protect me, the woman who came before. Gone was the woman who lived across the continent, who held the sources of my distress within her—at a distance. Now they were residing only in me, all too alive.

WHEN I WAS IN MY TWENTIES, they had a saying in the general press that "This is a generation without a future," referring to children born after World War II and in the wake of the explosion of the atomic bomb over Hiroshima and Nagasaki. It was assumed that we expected a bomb to go off at any moment. There would be a nuclear holocaust and that would be the end of the world. I remember thinking, "But I have always been without a future, and it is not because of the bomb." For I knew I had felt, since young, that I would not live long enough to have a future. I would not live to the next day or next year. Planning for it always seemed to me ridiculous. How could I count on that?

Since that time, I have been told in various psychotherapies that I seem not to maintain object constancy. When a person leaves me, I do not expect them back. I feel I have lost them forever. So it is hard for me to say goodbye even to casual acquaintances and even if the parting is brief. I have had to teach myself to say goodbye like other people do, as if it is something temporary, as if, of course, we will meet again, the other person will come back. Especially with intimates, including Hannah, particularly at first, I had to learn to say "Have a good time" in addition to "Goodbye." I had to recognize that Hannah might need permission to go away, to forget me for a while, to enjoy herself elsewhere. And that having her go with a feeling of guilt because she was leaving me was not a good idea. It was not useful to convey the sense of deep abandonment I felt. So I learned to say, "Have a good time," and Hannah learned to say, "I'll be back." Now with cell phones, I say, "Call me on your way home," and she does. It seems to make the leaving more about a return than not. It addresses my basic fear that when I am left, I will lose myself too, that my life will be over.

That I have always doubted I will have a future is something useful to remind myself as I worry about my writing and my nearing end. I have always had troublesome self-critical inner voices, I must tell myself, as I look at my writing or have my computer read it aloud and as I reflect, "Oh no, I can't do it. It's too revealing, too expressive of a dejected self, of myself not full of resourcefulness, not making an immediate positive sense of my dilemmas."

I find it helpful to remember that, years ago, when I first tried to write *Social Science and the Self*, I could not put my sentences together either, even as well as I can now. I had been awarded a grant to write about the unconventional approach I was pursuing in my academic work. I began writing a book-length monograph to expand on the "Fiction and Social Science" article I had written to accompany my lesbian community study, *The Mirror Dance*, to explain its unconventional "multiple-person" narrative style. I wanted to convey how constructed, how skillfully made up, even the very scientific tracts of social science were—that the line between fiction and social science was not clear. There were simply certain rules of social scientific fiction, some of which I had created in my own way in *The Mirror*

Dance. I was focusing on methodology, the underlying theory of knowledge involved. I wrote various chapters, enough in the end to comprise a short book, but I could not make sense of my sentences. I had to have a sociologist colleague as well as Hannah read my sentences repeatedly to tell me if they made sense, and if not, to offer suggestions for how to fix them. When I submitted the final manuscript to the foundation and to several publishers for review, I was amazed that anyone could read my sentences—that they were intelligible in a normal way. I have that book manuscript buried in my basement now in a box labeled "Susan's Academic Writings," but I have no desire to reread it.

More valuable to me are the personal stories I wrote in between my academic work that I dare not leave down in the basement where it is cold and damp but, instead, keep in two boxes on an upper shelf in my study closet. These are stories about my life that I did not view as sociology when I wrote them but that were, similarly, ways I sought significance in my experiences. A few of these stories have been published, but most remain private reminders of important relationships of my past. In my boxes, there is one novel, "Jenny's World," that I wrote after completing *The Mirror Dance*. I thought it was a good breather to write a novel after writing a study, that the personal writing complemented the academic. Initially, I intended this novel to be read by the psychotherapist I was seeing at the time because I felt I could not sit opposite her and tell her everything face-to-face. I wrote the novel in the third person, with Jenny representing me. My psychotherapist heard only the beginning of it when I read it aloud to her in several of our sessions, since she did not want to read outside the session. I wasn't sure how her reluctance to read would affect my motivation for my writing, but that mattered less, in the long run, than the fact that I found solace, comfort, and a sense of pride in getting my everyday life down in detail in "Jenny's World." In it, I described how I lived in the back room of the house of a woman with a son and a daughter, and how I identified with the boy and with living on the margins of someone else's life. I wrote about these intimate relationships of my past, seeking to experience them again.

When nine years later, I began writing *The Family Silver: Essays on Relationships among Women*, I found I could include a chapter from the novel in this collection. In this chapter, "Becoming a Lesbian," I had been able to speak very honestly about how I experienced my first deeply significant lesbian relationship. I could write more candidly, at that time, in the third person than I would have been able to do in the first person, describing what Fran, as I called her, meant to me that I might not have been able to say if I had to speak directly about myself. I could speak of my fears, my sense of loss, my sense of exuberance in now living with an older woman, a mature woman, my mother with me at last! I described Fran's naked woman's body and depicted us in bed and my own sexual feelings as I never would have been able to had I been writing more directly of myself. I developed a fondness for Jenny, for the other me, whom I could see and love when I had more distance and a less clear image of myself—the self I carry within as opposed to the self I can outwardly project and somehow better "see."

"Write your way out of it," I seemed to need to tell myself then, as perhaps I do now. "Jenny's World" was a way I could keep a positive sense of myself as I struggled with my internal silences. I would be able to do this later in *Things No Longer There* and *Traveling Blind*. But back when I wrote "Fiction and Social Science," I had too much internal confusion. Only after I sent the manuscript out for review did I have time to reflect back on why writing it had been so hard for me. It occurred to me that my frustration with my sentences may have been because during the time I was writing that monograph, my younger brother died. He committed suicide, we think, by standing or sitting on railroad tracks in Palo Alto and getting hit by a train. The same year, my psychotherapist stopped working because she had terminal cancer and she, too, died. When I considered that perhaps these two deaths were responsible for my inability to write in a manner that made sense to me, that recognition was extremely comforting. It wasn't me, it wasn't my failing, it was life getting me down. People have strong reactions to death, I thought. I was a person. Why not me? Yet I tend to believe that I should be impervious to such things. Particularly, I have always felt that my writing is a way I do not let the world get me down. It's my medicine, my working things out, my proof of my worth, my sanctuary. I cannot let it fail me. Yet sometimes it does. My mother's death, like that of my brother years ago, has crept in under my skin, I think, combining with negative attitudes I have internalized concerning aging, and with my inner vulnerabilities, affecting my ability to speak, to move from inner to outer, to have confidence in myself. I turn to my writing for relief and find it not there, and I wonder, will it ever be?

They say in the theater, "the show must go on." My father taught me to write every day. You got up, you lived and breathed, you ate, you wrote. This was his work, as now it is mine. My mother's work, in a way, was to churn inside, to have exalting inner forces, strong inner drives, and then to organize them with external order to command their settling down. If I have inherited her insides in some way, my own not as automatic and unseen as hers, if I have inherited her inner struggles, I believe I have also inherited her work—her need for that type of organizing activity that calms the outer surface, that commands the inner difficulties, the potentially self-defeating internal voices, and counters inner sadness. My writing, my talking to myself, my turning to psychotherapy and to intimate relationships—these are ways I try to calm things down, to speak back to the troublesome inner voices that threaten to undercut me. I work, too, at keeping physical order around me, in how I arrange things in my house, leaving clear surfaces as my mother did—to produce calm around her. But I doubt that my mother had as many self-critical inner voices as I do. I think she had deeply learned how to talk back to them, to avoid them or make them go away. She knew how to do that better than I do. I learned my self-critical voices from her—from her striking out and externalizing onto me the feelings of inadequacy or wrong she may otherwise have turned upon herself, and from being her daughter and feeling part of her.

I have got to get rid of these difficult voices. They are messing me up. They are lodged within me like an unwelcome guest running havoc in my house. They are a ball of yarn unraveling inside me, its strands going haywire. How can I get anything straight with this ball so tangled and taking up space, this emotional turbulence that is too often mine? Why do I now fear not so much that someone else will abandon me as that I will abandon myself? Have I become too isolated? I think perhaps I have. I know I have become too scared—too afraid of saying what is on my mind, afraid of exploring what is at the fore for me, admitting it, then using it, taking it somewhere, for first I have to face it.

My blindness is easier for me than my emotional dilemmas, more on the surface, not something I normally blame myself for. It doesn't go away, but it also does not torment. It is not an obstacle in the same way, though I find myself using similar words—to "overcome," proceed or persist in the face of it, not let it get me down. But my blindness is easier because there is more of a "me" present who can overcome, combat the blindness, pick up a cane or follow my dog, navigate, ask for help. There is a person at the center not letting it get her down. The problem with my inner emotional turmoil—my mother inside me, my inner struggles and self-doubt—is that it destroys the self. There is nobody there to combat the challenging forces, to confront or carry on, stand up, or move about. I feel stuck. Where is my motivation to come from? Then I think of what I need to take care of—feed my cats, walk with my guide dog Teela, play with my pet dog Esperanza. I need to brush my teeth. I take care of the outer shell—of my relationships with others and with myself. I turn to Hannah, who is an extraordinarily positive presence for me, who helps me feel valued and cared for. We have dinner together, we talk about the day, we help each other out—our small interactions bringing me much joy.

I often wonder why I have my difficulties, and I tend to blame them on my mother. But I know that the cause is more complex and, indeed, less important than the fact that I live with this internal churning, this threat to myself, and with a sense that I must constantly conceal my inner struggles.

Because I am always hiding these struggles and trying to pass as similar to others who seem to have less inner strife than I do, I constantly feel there is a great difference between myself and others. I seek to bridge the gap between us with my writing, creating a kind of intimacy that is often hard for me face-to-face. Through repeated practice, I have developed a certain skill at it, a fluency. It is like another language that I am constantly teaching and reteaching myself, an inner language full of surprises. Without this intimate narrative, my inner talking to myself, I could not achieve the outer— my adventures, my steps forward. It is a basic survival mechanism for me. Yet exposing my inner talking—letting others know some of what goes into it—is not easy for me, particularly exposing the negative aspects, the problems I seek to overcome. I fear becoming defeated by them, or making readers feel defeated and like they have to pull away from me. Yet usually I find that when I speak honestly of myself, other people feel I am speaking of something they also find within. Perhaps they feel like outsiders, too, who must strive to conform and who have similar hidden battles with self-worth.

I think the world is full of a conventional surface, of common conversation—what is acceptable to say, the shared language, the shared constructed experience. The purpose of my kind of writing— of intimate narrative—is to be honest, to break through, go beneath that conventional surface, speak the vulnerability, the inner forces, the inner stream of thought, the consciousness not usually talked about that is there nonetheless.

In my writing, I experiment with words, trying again and again to feel free from constraints, to get that sense of adventure, of value, of creating something worthwhile out of the swirl of everything. I wonder whether I will ever again be the girl on the horse with the curly hair, so happy, riding off. Yet with each glimpse, I am her. I am not in the past, I am in the present, which requires more resourcefulness than I ever would have imagined. It requires that I open myself up, that I admit to emotional difficulties, talk back to the negative inner voices.

I REMEMBER THAT WHEN I USED TO DRIVE, I would sometimes take the car down the coast from San Francisco south toward Año Nuevo, and as I drove west and caught a view of the ocean, I would suddenly feel free. I would be happy, thinking aloud, wondering what my thoughts were, wondering if one of them would be a new piece of writing. I would be inspired from the sheer motion of it, the open air, the sea, the sense that I was on my own. I would be happy in those moments, adventurous, optimistic, all troubles would fade. It didn't matter that I had inner difficulties because I had these exhilarating moments. I would think about something new I was going to write; I would bring back shells or sand dollars. I would have lunch at Duarte's Tavern, visit the marsh where I went after my brother died to remember him and how he liked the small town of Pescadero.

My moments of adventure come in other ways for me now, since I cannot drive anymore. Often I have them when walking with Teela, who happily leads me, her confidence contagious. As we stride forward quickly, even on city streets, the motion is invigorating, with me looking up at the sky, taking in the air, Teela with her nose forward, ears back. Motion seems necessary to those freeing moments, movement that quiets the inner forces, that opens up new vistas, a sense of being alone, but not totally alone—going off, able to come back. I have those moments walking with my cherished dog. They are not gone. Perhaps the walking is a way not to sit, not to brood. I must concentrate on my direction, on getting from here to there. But most of it is automatic, so there is time to think. I am then the teenaged girl with curly hair. The horse is gold not chestnut brown. The sky is bright, sometimes a hill. I need more of those moments now, moments for the new dreams, the new story I am going to write, the new places to go, the next trip to New Mexico when I will be using my camera—a substitute for my eyes. When I will use my inner vision, my sense of what I might see, hoping to see not inner trouble or lack of worth, but something that glows—my mother's bracelet, the shine of silver, the positive passed down, the escape, the way into a future full of light and new dreams.

I think that reviewer's comment that she wished to be me meant so much to me because it reminded me of my sense of adventure. Her comment made me feel valued and that I could escape my doldrums if only I would focus on the adventures I was taking or could take, if only I saw myself in terms of, "What new possibility can I embark on today and how can it reward me?"

I am grateful for that reviewer's comment, though I cannot find it online anymore. Possibly it is no longer there. She was somewhere in the Midwest, perhaps Iowa. I cannot find her discussion, but I remember her words, that sentence. It has come to mind recently as I seek to confront my fears and it has been of more help than I ever could have known. I would like to find the woman who wrote it and thank her. So often I have grave self-doubts. And then her sentence comes to mind, "I want to be Susan Krieger." And then I challenge myself: If someone else wants to be me, why not me?

April 2012

Part IV

Seeking Connection

TWELVE

---◆◆◆◆◆---

The Art of the Intimate Narrative

I AM A SOCIOLOGIST AND A FEMINIST ETHNOGRAPHER. I write studies that focus on particular experiences in order to contribute to broader social knowledge. In some of my studies, I have interviewed and focused on the lives of others; in other studies, I have drawn from my own personal experiences. In both cases, I have been committed to experimenting with narrative form, presenting data in an innovative way by creating a portrait of a social reality that is direct, vivid, complex, and intimate and that takes the reader on a journey—weaving a way through a situation in order to get to know it. Traditionally, sociological narratives are written with a tone of objectivity and superior authority, with theoretical generalizations subsuming the presentation of specific data, and with a narrative voice that commands respect because of its distanced and formal vantage point and familiar legitimating style. I have been affected deeply by the social science tradition within sociology; at the same time, I view myself as an innovator within that field.

In this chapter, I revisit my studies published in the past thirty years, reflecting on a process of creating different and more personal narrative forms. *Come, Let Me Guide You* clearly extends the themes of my prior work concerning community, gender, identity, and blindness, and it takes a step further in the tenderness of its approach. I hope that my discussion of my writing as it has evolved toward increasing intimacy will encourage others who also seek to speak with a unique voice in a chosen field.

WHY I WRITE

WHEN I READ OVER MY PUBLISHED WORK, I am particularly struck by those places where my individual voice—my inner, unabashed, vernacular, sometimes embarrassing voice—comes through. I am amazed that my inner ways of speaking have made it to the printed page and recorded word. I feel proud when I find my vernacular inner voice arguing for personal expression, as, for example, in my initial methodological work, *Social Science and the Self:* "I knew I would have to 'assert myself,' even if my assertion felt uncomfortable, and even if I would continually feel I was illegitimately imposing myself on my data. . . . I decided, 'I must write about what I can relate to. I must write a personal account.'" The continuity of my desire for a personal voice is clear in my next book, *The Family Silver,* in which I wrote that "because these essays draw on my internal emotional life and deal with issues of sexual preference, they result in a study that is intimate far beyond my prior works, and beyond what is usually found in the social sciences and considered acceptable in academic discourse. The intimacy of the essays is their central challenge." Still, I am shocked by the many personal revelations that appear in my subsequent ethnography, *Things No Longer There,* where, in a story about a meaningful past relationship, I wrote:

> *She took my hand quietly and led me to sit beside her. She held me close and kissed me. I kissed her back. She rested her head back on the couch for a moment. Then she held me to her even more tightly and cried, her large tears rolling slowly down her cheeks. "My deep river flows only for you," she said. I said nothing and let myself be held, fearing her feelings for me would go away.*

The intimacy of my work is pivotal for me. I am a very private, often isolated person—a writer at the heart of my being a sociologist—although the title "writer" is still hard for me to accept, because

I have long thought it means someone frivolous who cannot quite earn enough money to make a living. My father was a writer. My mother often worried that he would not earn enough or have a stable enough income. But I seem to have copied him, his habits of waking early, writing first thing in the morning, writing almost every morning. It's as if the day is wasted, as if there's nothing there if I don't write, which, for me, means to think, to contemplate, to get at my deepest feelings, to put something down, to have it out. It means to imagine, to invent, to inhabit a fantasy world where everyone appreciates my thoughts, honors my perspective, says "Wow!," finds me there in my chair writing or at my computer—an unsung talent, a woman of value to be cherished, applauded, and held close.

Gone is the isolation as I sit alone in my study, gone is the fear, the anxiety. I am focusing only on the work, on putting my thoughts and feelings together, articulating, looking for insights, sailing away on the emotions involved, trying not to destroy these emotions, not to change them, not to stray from what seems to me true or accurate, what was actually present in a situation: a lesbian community or a hippie rock radio station I studied, a feminist classroom I wrote about, my own inner responses to my blindness—all of these subjects of my studies. I fear greatly, as I write, that I'll misrepresent others or myself, get wrong the name of an out-of-business gas station in a desert town I pass through in *Traveling Blind*. I fear that if I don't "get it right," people will know, and then they won't trust me or my work. They'll put it down, decide the narrator is unreliable. What else might she have gotten wrong? My deep concern is to be a reliable narrator, to provide a compelling read, but not by shocking or misleading the reader. My fear of getting it wrong is shaped by the truth-seeking norms of the social sciences. These norms guide even my intimate writing. They influence my choice of subject, my way of obtaining evidence, the way I organize my portraits, my sense of faithfulness to sources and to the "truth" of a situation that I seek to represent.

When I write, I am always involved in a relationship with the reader, with many readers actually—all those who figure in my mind, and who, I imagine, will appreciate me, or who I hope will, and with some who won't, who are questioning me all the time: Have you got it right? Is that true? Are you telling me what I need to know? Have you prepared me for what is about to happen before it occurs—for example, when you were hit by that car as you crossed the street, did you tell me first that you failed to see it coming because of your lack of sight? Have you described your emotions in the proper order, the order in which they occurred? Have you figured out the mileage correctly between Deming and Lordsburg? Have you interpreted fairly the words of the woman who spoke to you in the Mimbres General Store? Have you intellectually made sense of your experiences and created generalizations that are not hasty but true? If so, you've done the best you can for the moment. Then on to the next moment.

Many of these internal questions emerge from my early methodological training in the social sciences, which emphasized veracity about people and places represented. That training also encouraged cautious and multidimensional theoretical views of a subject and, above all, required that assertions about "what is out there" be put through repeated tests. My desire to be faithful to the realities I describe in my work might have emerged on its own, but probably not as strongly. I am not a writer of fiction, nor of topical nonfiction. Rather, I am always somehow "structuring a study," using my writing as a tool to help me know, and using myself in the service of creating a larger portrait of a complex social reality—a portrait that can enhance others' understandings as well.

Initially in doing the research for my studies, I exclusively interviewed others. Over time, however, I came to want to say things or to explore aspects of situations about which others could not easily tell me. I began to probe my own experiences of lesbianism, gender, blindness, and identity to get at hidden complexities that seemed to me important to articulate and document. I began to write a personal feminist version of ethnography, drawing on a female, often understated and vulnerable inner voice, not the traditional authoritative sociological narrative style, but a personal style increasingly comfortable for me and one that gave me a sense of accomplishment.

MY EVOLVING STYLE

I USED TO WRITE POETRY when I was in graduate school. I used the pen name Sarah Kistler, who never actually published anything. But I thought that my poetry was too revealing, too embarrassing, not something for an academic to have appear under her name. Often after I wrote a poem that I thought was especially good, I would feel I had to leave my house because the truth in it, what I said, even if only in a few words—for my poems were short and intimate—felt too powerful, too plain-spoken, too exposed. I had to leave the house to get away from my words.

Back when I wrote poetry as my main form of expression, I remember being told by members of a writing group that my poetry wasn't really poetry. It was too prosy, too simple. Of course, it did not rhyme, but it also lacked the usual conventions of poetry such as metaphors. I thought that the people who criticized me just did not understand. They were old-fashioned, traditional, liking the standard forms of poetry, affected, not plain-spoken like me, not as advanced as me. These are very superior attitudes, but I had them, perhaps self-protectively. Back then, when I was getting to know a person as a potential friend, my test of them, my way of having them get to know me, was to bring a folder of my poetry for them to read. If they responded well, I felt they knew me, and I then felt more secure with them. I felt accepted and special.

As it has turned out, my academic writing has become an extension of my earlier personal poetry, and like that poetry, it is plain-spoken, though the plainness is deceptive, hiding much intellectual thought and complex self-consciousness lying just beneath the surface. I did not start out intentionally to write poetry in academic clothing, but over the years, my writing has become more intimate, more emotional and personal, as my desire to speak from an individual standpoint has deepened. Although always innovative in style and concerned with cadences, rhythms, and interior truths, my writing has become more relaxed and self-accepting over time, I think, as I develop new skills and take on new challenges with each new study. Like my early poetry, my academic writing continues to be direct, often colloquial, and seemingly lacking in artifice. By the latter, I mean that my style seems to be quite natural, especially when I write in the first person. The naturalness of the style of expression, however, belies the work that goes into it. I often wish I could write that naturally or smoothly initially, but my personal voice is actually the result of much self-conscious thinking and multiple revisions as I work on crafting both the persona of who I am as I speak and the words that go into each ethnographic portrait.

The words, my father used to tell me, should disappear. They should seem not to be there, not to call attention to themselves. As I craft each study, I concentrate on the central subject or theme—lesbianism, gender, blindness, identity—and I work at having my words slip away, guiding the reader through my content, making it acceptable. The writing, I tell myself, should make the content go down like a smooth chilled oyster suddenly sliding down the back of one's throat before it's clear whether, in fact, this was something one wanted to eat. As I write, I seek to move the reader quickly through my text, discouraging stops. I want the reader to feel right there with me—in my thoughts, my feelings, sharing my observations, having my emotions in the process of having hers. I try to smooth the path, stir feelings, prompt new insights. I feel less alone as I engage with the reader, and I hope that the reader, too, will feel less alone. My desire to bring the reader with me has continued through a variety of books, each with a different subject matter and setting, and each posing a different challenge for me, prompting me to create, in each case, a new and fitting narrative form.

My first two ethnographies were third-person narratives—*Hip Capitalism,* an organizational study of a hippie rock radio station emerging in the Summer of Love in San Francisco that traced the station's cooptation into mainstream corporate America, and *The Mirror Dance,* a study of a midwestern lesbian community and how individuals sought and found personal identity within it. In both of these books, I drew from interviews I had conducted to create unusual narratives that conveyed the thoughts and feelings of individuals. The style of *Hip Capitalism* was extremely novelistic for sociology, developing individual characters and a drama evocative of the hippie 1960s. The narrative structure I created in *The Mirror Dance* broke further with convention in that it was composed entirely of the voices of the women of the lesbian community responding to and commenting upon one another in a "multiple-person stream-of-consciousness" fashion, without an omniscient authorial voice. The study provided a "bird's-eye view," like overhearing the gossip of a small town. In the introduction, I explained that: "*The Mirror Dance* is clearly an experiment, both in women's language and in social science method. It is composed of an interplay of voices that echo, again and again, themes of self and community, sameness and difference, loss and change."

Although the narrative structure of *The Mirror Dance* worked out well in the end, it did not come readily to me. For two years after I completed my interviews, I could not write up my findings or figure out how to interpret my data. I picked up my interview notes, put them down, carried them across the country with me to a new university job, unable to identify significant themes or ideas with which to understand what the women had told me. Only when I developed an exercise for "re-engaging" with my original interview experiences and my period of involvement as a member of the lesbian community did I begin to find a voice with which to speak back to the voices of the women and to understand their struggles. Reflecting on my own experiences, I found themes of likeness and difference, merger and separation, and processes of losing and finding a sense of self that helped me also to interpret other members of the community.

In an article titled, "Beyond 'Subjectivity': The Use of the Self in Social Science," I wrote about my process of drawing from within myself to arrive at insights also useful for understanding others. That article was a turning point for me in terms of method and led to my subsequent book-length study, *Social Science and the Self: Personal Essays on an Art Form*. In both these works, I spoke personally, arguing that the self of the inquirer, rather than being viewed as a contaminant that would detrimentally bias a study, could more fruitfully be viewed as a source of knowledge that can make a study more true. "The great danger of doing injustice to the reality of the 'other,'" I suggested, "does not come about through use of the self, but through lack of use of a full enough sense of self, which, concomitantly, produces a stifled, artificial, limited, and unreal knowledge of others."

After speaking personally in "Beyond 'Subjectivity'" and *Social Science and the Self*, I found that I could not go back to my earlier third-person style. A self-reflective approach to research and writing had become too rewarding, too rich a source of insights for me. This is not to say that I found a personal approach easier, for I would soon discover that it posed many new challenges and required new goals. For my approach to be valuable, I thought, it would have to generate insights not easily gained in other ways, and that were often not as obvious to others as they were to me. It would require that I achieve a level of honesty and self-reliance unequaled in my prior work, often pushing myself to say what was difficult, and it would require that I stand up, even more than before, to the naysayers and critics.

For just as my earlier poetry had been criticized as "not really poetry," I soon found that critics questioned whether my sociological work was "really social science." I think this was because, even when written in the third person, my studies specifically presented intimate details drawn from individuals' lives, rather than relying on a more traditional sociological style in which abstract theories and hypotheses—or generalizations—subsumed the details. Each of my ethnographies, instead, provided a complex, multifaceted narrative portrait. This portrait was my organizing device, or interpretation, with theory implicit. My authorial voice was understated and often invisible in my early studies, sometimes intensely personal in the later ones, opening up a complexity rather than summarizing it. It was a narrative voice far different from that of a traditional male authoritative speaker. I invited the reader to join with me in each setting, becoming part of a community or adventure, experiencing it with me, drawing her own conclusions while considering mine.

NEW INTIMATE NARRATIVES

AFTER *SOCIAL SCIENCE AND THE SELF*, my next three books extended my method into new realms. In *The Family Silver: Essays on Relationships among Women*, I focused on the invisible worlds that women create and on the hidden wealth—the female cultures and customs, the "family silver"—that women pass on to one another. More candidly self-reflective in style than I had been before, in *The Family Silver* I drew on my experiences as a lesbian within academia as well as outside. I looked closely at women's intimate ties, the ambiguities of female gender roles, and the risks of academic nonconformity. "In previous work," I explained, "I have studied others, and it seems to me that it is far easier to look at others and think one sees what is occurring than to look at oneself and try to see themes, explanations, interpretations, to offer stories that are both true and acceptable. When one looks at oneself, the picture becomes more complex, more intimate. The easy answers disappear." In a chapter on gender roles, I especially confronted this challenge of suggesting social complexity through individual self-reflection. For example:

People who know me, for instance, think I look like myself, and that I am a woman. My clothes seem fitting to me. They are not aware of how much I feel, and fear, I am a man. When younger and wanting so much to be a man—in order to be free of being a woman, or like my mother, and in order simply to be free—I used to take greater pride in being mistaken for a man than I do now, and to feel less discomforted when called one. Maybe I got so accustomed to the pants and freedom that being called a man did not seem so much of a compliment anymore. I felt better when seen as a woman. But maybe the reason has more to do with a change in what the genders came to stand for in my particular world. At some point, the meanings switched, and good became female, and freedom became female, and so did I.

Gender and lesbian themes persisted into my next study, *Things No Longer There: A Memoir of Losing Sight and Finding Vision,* where I began to explore issues of inner sight. I had found that my experiences of "moving on and growing older" led to losses that I needed to confront. I was interested in how, although the outer world may change over time and old relationships and landscapes disappear, inner visions of them persist, giving meaning, jarring the senses with a very different, and often more valuable, picture than what appears before the eyes. To create my narrative in *Things No Longer There,* I drew from my inner imagery, painting pictures from memory of special places I had known that were now built over with new homes and roads, and of intimate personal relationships of my past now gone in the outer world but still very present in my mind. I sought to suggest that vision, very importantly, is made up of such inner imagery, extending the limits of visual sight and rich with emotional meanings.

I wrote, too, of my recent experience of losing my eyesight and of how, when objects in the outer world "literally became no longer visible to me," I began to need not only to use my mind to see what my eyes did not, but also "to create a counterposing internal vision so that my sense of my own value would remain intact." In the face of many external attitudes that might make me feel that my loss of eyesight rendered me less valuable as a person, I needed to develop an alternate, positive inner vision—a view of myself as different and still capable, rather than as diminished by my lack of sight. In *Things No Longer There*, I was committed to revealing the importance of such inner rebuilding and of retaining crucial memories from the past despite a sense of loss. In stories about blindness, lesbianism, and emotional connection, I wrote more intimately about myself in all the portraits in that book than I had before.

Interestingly, when *Things No Longer There* required a subtitle, the publisher suggested using the term "memoir." At first I was taken aback, since I viewed my book as a study organized around the theme of valuing inner vision when outer landscapes disappear. However, I knew that the purpose was to identify the work in a popular category that would be useful for sales representatives in selling the book to bookstores. What I did not at first realize was how much the word memoir would soon haunt me, and not only because it appeared in my title. Increasingly as I began to use a more intimate narrative style—moving from reflecting on the lives of others to exploring my own experiences in my ethnographies—I found that I often was perceived as "writing memoir." Although not necessarily a criticism, this categorization felt like a slight to me, or at least a misunderstanding. In my mind, I was still using an approach deeply affected by my early training in social science research methodology. I was committed to faithfulness and to structuring my narratives to illumine social realities. I used my personal experiences selectively to that end. A close look at my narratives reveals, I think, a deliberately detailed structure that is more like a presentation of data than it is like the more autobiographical form of memoir, which relies on conventional expectations of storyline and personal drama.

The themes I introduced in *Things No Longer There* concerning blindness and sight became further elaborated in my subsequent ethnography, *Traveling Blind: Adventures in Vision with a Guide Dog by My Side*, where I focused specifically on mobility. What is it like to "travel blind"? I asked. What is it like to live in an ambiguous world—as I was beginning to do—where things are not black and white so much as present and absent, shades of gray? What is it like to navigate through constantly changing external imagery that requires changing inner perspectives as well? What is it like to travel with a guide dog, to have an invisible disability? What can experiences of blindness tell us about sight?

In *Traveling Blind*, I explored, as well, the gratitude I felt in sharing my path with my intimate partner, Hannah, making the book a romance, as well as a story about my changing perceptions as I navigated the world with my new guide dog, Teela. As the three of us travel through the Southwest, I often use desert imagery to help me examine issues of blindness and sight. The book is full of descriptions of vast skies, mountains, and mesas, often seen imperfectly, and of my internal responses to them as I attempt to arrive at insights of broader usefulness. "Like the desert that gradually reclaims its own," I reflected, "my vision has a quality of gradual change in which my efforts to see—to grasp what is before me, and to appreciate my experiences in a positive way—count more than my losses." And "the comfort I viewed in the landscape was, in part, because my blindness lent a softness to the scenery, blending the trees and fields together. Sometimes I yearned for clarity, for the individual tree shapes to stand out, but I also accepted the softness as a gift of my blindness."

In this unusually focused travel narrative, I wished to take the reader with me on my journeys even more than before—through airports and city streets as well as desert towns, using my personal experiences to create broader understandings. As I described what I saw and did not see, I sought to present vision as a multidimensional achievement in which touch, sound, smell, mind, and feeling count as much as visual sight and to suggest that the blind also see—through a mixture of these senses, through adaptation, intuition, and through living in the world of the sighted.

I think that in *Traveling Blind*, as in my prior works, I was again pushing a recognition of something hard to see—an invisible reality. In *Things No Longer There* and *The Family Silver*, lesbianism was the central invisible reality that I had focused upon, seeking to describe it in an underlying way for what I felt it was—a difference, something soft and at my center of great import in my life, but for which I often did not have the words to describe it well, to acknowledge it, to "see" it. Like blindness, lesbianism felt so connected to my vulnerable inner sense of self and comfort that I felt it was difficult to reveal, for fear of adverse consequences.

Drawing from my experiences to describe invisible realities has often left me feeling very exposed in my narratives, wondering: Will others like me? Will they see what I see? Will they believe me? Will my prose carry the reader along as I wish? Am I being too intimate? Not intimate enough? In my sociological writing, as in my life, I am extremely sensitive to public exposure and to the negative judgments it may bring, as suggested in this passage, from the "Airport Stories" chapter of *Traveling Blind*, about my navigating with Teela:

Airports—they are so very public and I am so very private, and so obvious with Teela. I feel odd being guided by a dog, trying to do it in good form yet looking like I'm blind. I am unsure of what others see, unsure of what I see myself,

*doubtful inside of who I am, and of what I should be doing
all the while as I am doing it, as Teela pulls me forward and
I follow her. She weaves me through the other passengers, the
world whizzes by me out of focus and I wonder, am I doing
it right, am I blind enough? Do I need this dog? But if I let
go of Teela's harness for even a moment, if I lose her, she then
turns back and looks strangely at me, as if to say, "Where are
you? You're supposed to be on the other end of this." I pick up
the harness handle and start again the rolling walk we share.*

Now, in *Come, Let Me Guide You: A Life Shared with a Guide
Dog*, I further explore the importance of my relationship with Teela,
extending themes concerning blindness, intimacy, gender, and identity introduced in my prior work. In writing these stories about
our life together, I have found that examining my relationship with
Teela has led me not only to new recognitions about myself and
others, but also to new and deepening possibilities for intimate
expression. In speaking of a time when Teela became injured, for
example, I reflect:

*In that moment, and in others like it, I have had to realize
how deeply Teela's life had become intertwined with mine.
As she breathes, I do; when she is injured, I hurt. When she
is happy, I glow with her joy. It's an odd bond, an unusual
bond—no guide in life is different, no relationship less importantly tended than this one has been for me. Teela has been a
guide to a new way in the world for me, much needed because
of my loss of sight; a guide to getting older, and a guide to
sharing my life. In the nine and-a-half years I have had her,
she has been with me almost every place I have gone. When
I have had to leave her behind, I have missed her. I have run
after her when she has strayed, listened for her tinkling collar,*

played with her, worked with her, watched her sleep, traveled
in cabs and in snowy forests with her, kept her clean and safe,
and tried to share her dreams.

Writing intimate narratives may not seem the best thing to do
for someone who tends to hide, to fear what others may think, who
tends to feel unacceptable. Yet this writing always has been healing
for me, clarifying, giving light and air to something deep within. It
has enabled me to write it out, present it to the world, feel present,
assess where I am now, who I am, sift through the complexities of
the various experiences in which I participate and observe. For me,
there is a great treasure trove everywhere of things to see and know,
to describe, to interpret as I seek to hold onto and cherish what I
have lived. Those special moments, special experiences felt intensively within, are often difficult to articulate to the outer world, but
always worth the trying.

I was pleased to represent the lesbian community in *The Mirror
Dance;* finally to get the hippie rock radio station's story down in its
period-piece detail in *Hip Capitalism;* to "write myself in" in *Social
Science and the Self.* I was then shocked and delighted to be able
to continue to have my inner thoughts, my colloquial yet crafted
stream-of-consciousness way of getting at underlying realities,
appear again on the printed page in four successive ethnographic
works probing issues of gender, blindness, and identity. Each book
has extended the reach of my intimacies. In each, I have combined
the norms of a social science with the practice of an introspective art.

In the future, I hope to explore more of what I see beneath the
surface of social experiences. I remain committed to writing intimately, to drawing from within myself to achieve broader insights.
Giving myself internal permission to represent reality "as I see it,"
however, is a difficult thing to do, especially, perhaps, because I am
a woman—taught early on not to emphasize or call attention to

myself, taught that the personal, the particularly individual may not be worth much. Flying in the face of that sense of lack of worth, I pick up my pen or sit at my computer, trying to set forth the words, hoping to catch that glimmer, that flow of inner thought and feeling that will create insights, a sense of knowing, of feeling I was here. Then tentatively, each time I finish a study, when I get enough of that stream-of-consciousness out, enough of my inner sense of experience, I offer it to readers to learn what they will say. At that moment, with each new study, I am back again all too easily to my days in graduate school when I gingerly took out a folder with my poems in it to show to a new potential friend. Would she like me? Would she read them? Would I be acceptable, applauded, cherished, and held close?

September 2010 and July 2014

THIRTEEN

$\bullet\!\bullet\!\!\!\!\bullet\!\!\!\!\blacklozenge\!\!\!\!\bullet\!\!\!\!\bullet\!\!\!\!\bullet$

Women and Disabilities

I REMEMBER THE FIRST TIME I taught my course on women and disabilities. To prepare the syllabus, I went into the campus bookstore to look for readings I might use. Back then, I could still make out the titles of books on shelves, for the eye condition causing my blindness had not yet progressed as far as it later would. I looked for a disabilities section. There was none. I looked under health and found some titles, then under personal essay collections, women's studies, and self-help. I faced a dilemma: What of all the possible maladies besetting women should I consider to be disabilities? Was breast cancer a disability? What about mental illness? The array of health problems, the diseases and conditions that women might acquire—such as multiple sclerosis, diabetes, chronic fatigue, arthritis—overwhelmed me and seemed too varied for me to comprehend. I decided I would include only those conditions I felt were most closely suggested by the blue and white icon that stood for disabled access—a wheelchair with a stick figure of a person sitting in it. I would not include cancer or mental illness, two subjects that, frankly, scared me. There has to be some way to determine what is in the category and not, I thought. Then I began to teach the course.

The history of teaching my Women and Disabilities seminar over the past twelve years has been a story of expanding my original categories of what is considered to be a disability and of accepting many of the conditions that I first excluded. It has been a story of my becoming more brave in what I have been willing to take on, and of my students becoming more brave, as they, and I, have sought to confront our prejudices, stereotypes, and fears; it has also been an adventure in sharing my intimate narrative approach with the students and encouraging them to apply some of the methods that inform my own writing. Over the years that I have taught the course, I have gained important personal insights about my blindness, my inner emotional life, and my interdependence with others—expanding from a place of little knowledge to more profound understandings. Throughout, I have been drawn to new recognitions by the generous contributions of the students.

In teaching this course, I assign readings that are almost exclusively first-person accounts by disabled women. I supplement these by asking the students to interview disabled women weekly and to reflect on disability or disability-like experiences of their own. From the start of each quarter, I am intent on breaking down an us/them distinction that the students arrive with and that often accompanies my subject—that between disabled and nondisabled. In our first class session, I ask the students to discuss: "If you could choose, what disability would you like to have?" And, "Would you rather be born with that disability or come to it later in life?" Answering these questions, they are immediately in the disabled camp, and I feel less alone in the classroom.

The seminar has numbered between four and twelve students each year. The majority are premed students majoring in human biology with a women's health concentration. They are taking the course to become better doctors. A few are Feminist Studies majors, reflecting the program in which I teach. Only one or two students each term come to the course self-identified as disabled. Sometimes none of the students identify this way. The small number of disabled students choosing this elective course is, in part, a result of the greater risk perceived by them, since in their coursework, disabled students often seek to escape the separateness and stigma associated with disabilities. They may also be concerned about becoming the focus of others' attention and judgment.

That my disabilities seminar is small in size should not surprise me, but it always does. I used to teach a course titled Women and Organizations, where the classroom overflowed with the initial turnout and I had to select among the students to limit the size. It is as if teaching Women and Disabilities is just the opposite, as if one course were implicitly about "women and success" and the other "women and failure." I don't think that is so, but I do think the stigma associated with disabilities and the desire to avoid having a disability have a discouraging effect, and I often wish to counteract that. One advantage of the small class size, however, is that the students and I can sit closely around the seminar table, creating our own private world.

To describe that world, I draw here on the students' voices as well as my own, using quotations from papers submitted in the course in the spring quarter of 2011, a year when I had an unusually articulate group of students. I have assigned pseudonyms and protected individual identities yet sought to remain faithful to each student's original meanings. Interweaving the students' voices with mine, I trace the course experience week to week, focusing on insights gained and the use of personal narratives as a route to learning. Although this account reflects one term in the teaching of the course, the themes and topics are those that have persisted through the decade. I wrote this description immediately after teaching the course that spring, eager to share what, for me, has been cumulatively a life-altering experience and transformative for the students as well. The classroom environment has been important to this learning. As one student reflected:

Having this small of a class was new to me but it was a welcome change. With a smaller number of students in the class, it is easier not only to have your share of time talking with the class but also provides the opportunity to really get to know each student on a personal level. Both the students and the teacher actually share a relationship that goes beyond a grade on a paper. I also felt that with the small classroom came a safe environment where everyone could say their thoughts and not expect to be shot down nor attacked but just listened to and given an honest opinion back. (Mary Beth)

In this intimate seminar, I ask the students to speak personally in class and in their writings. They submit weekly papers in which they discuss their feelings as well as their thoughts in response to the readings and research. I encourage them to be honest and not to fear expressing prejudices and negative stereotypes concerning disabilities, since I feel that, if unexpressed, their underlying emotions can get in the way of their learning. I tell them that I, too, have internalized many negative and rejecting attitudes toward disabilities and that it is unavoidable in our culture. Initially and throughout the quarter, I draw on my own disability experiences in class discussions, trying to provide an example of self-reflection for the students to follow. In my assignments, I pose guiding questions and repeatedly ask the students to consider how female gender affects the authors we read, the women they interview, and their own experiences. The class is often composed only of women, although in some instances, I have had one or two men. I ask the male students to look at female qualities within themselves that perhaps are often denied. The students each choose an individual research topic to explore in depth during the quarter to help focus their learning.

Each year that I have taught this course, I have noticed that the students come to it with a central question of their own that often surprises me. That is, "How should I treat a disabled person so as not to offend her or him?" This question is raised in our very first class session, and the students go out with it in the end, as if the next disabled person they meet after our course is over will be the test of their learning. "Will I now know what to say? And if I don't know, will I be more comfortable with not knowing?" they wonder. There goes all my work in breaking down the us/them dichotomy, I feel. Or possibly not. For I hope that a sense of being part of "them" will linger with the students long after our course is over, so that in facing a woman in a wheelchair, a blind woman, a woman with a chronic illness, a student will feel, "I know you a little. I can reach into myself and address you. I can say something. I am not as much of a fool as I thought I was. And you can always correct me. I have broken the ice. My teacher said the worst thing I can do is be silent, not acknowledge another disabled person, not speak, not be interested, not care." Or at least these are things I would like the students to remember. I think they definitely will feel more at ease in relation to disabled people and possibly more accepting of disabilities within themselves.

> *One thing that I feel I have accomplished over the quarter is being more comfortable in talking about women and disability, especially when it comes to the language that I use surrounding the subject. I remember at the very beginning of the quarter, I was very careful, and almost uncomfortable, about the language that I was choosing to use in my papers. (Sylvia)*

I organize my course syllabus with guiding topic headings for each week to reflect themes I have found important in studying the lives of disabled women. The introductory week's title is "Women's Psychological as Well as Physical Health" to suggest that we will be focusing on disabled women's inner perceptions of their health rather than on medical definitions. I tell the students that I think different issues emerge when studying women's experiences with disabilities than they may be familiar with from general conversations that tend to be legalistic and concerned with rights, eligibility, categorization, degree of disability, and ideas of independence. In studying women, I explain, I find that the issues become more personally intimate. Experiences of invisibility are prominent, and the "hidden work" that disabled women engage in is highlighted, particularly the hidden emotional work of camouflaging their disabilities.

In the first class, I try to convey to the students that I think women are strong and entrepreneurial in the face of disabilities, that they rarely sacrifice their caretaking of others for their own self-care, and that I think women, in a way, know the world through disability—through limitation, weakness, vulnerability, complexity, adaptation, and through doing more while being valued less. These gender attributes may be social constructs, but they are quite real. I think women have complex and wonderful inner emotional lives that the study of disabilities unearths. There are, of course, hardships and distresses unequally shared by the genders—such as poverty, discrimination, and lack of equal regard—but the emphasis in my course is not on an accounting but, rather, on learning to see and appreciate how women uniquely experience disabilities. How do disabled women see the world and themselves? In my view, understanding their experiences may help us to address broader issues of acknowledging diversity and meeting human needs.

These initial themes recur in the second week, on "The Diversity of Women's Experiences of Disability, Hidden Disabilities, and What Difference Does Female Gender Make?" The students begin readings and write their first papers. Our readings, by women of varied ages and sociocultural backgrounds, address cerebral palsy, multiple sclerosis, learning disabilities, deafness, and environmental disability. Two overview articles place the field of Feminist Disability

Studies within a broader academic context. Our main text, Nancy Mairs' *Waist-High in the World: A Life among the Nondisabled*, is an unusually candid and insightful account of disability through Mairs' experiences with multiple sclerosis.

In class, we often discuss how disabilities are socially constructed. The idea that a disability is a product of attitudes and institutions that disable, rather than strictly of a physical or medical condition, is new to some of the students. One example they find helpful is that it is not the physiological limitations of a woman in a wheelchair that makes her disabled when crossing a street but the fact that there are curbs. In their writing, the students begin speaking personally about their responses to the readings:

> *I love Nancy Mairs' writing style so much because she actually speaks to the reader, engaging us, asking us to do things such as when she asks us to look around from a seated position, explaining that that is how she views the world everyday, waist–high but knee–deep. (Mary Beth)*

> *The article written by Megan Jones, along with the other articles that address invisible disabilities, made me feel guilty. Before learning about these unseen disabilities, I have always believed that people with disabilities must have some form of obvious deformity. . . . I am often suspicious of people who park in handicapped parking spaces who look "normal." And normal to me simply means that the person is capable of walking, seeing, hearing; is young; drives a nice car; and wears nice clothes. It is as if I could only understand disability at its extreme case scenario. After reading these articles, I feel awful that I have made these judgments. It is difficult enough to live with a disability, let alone have to prove it to others. (Joanna)*

*One of the articles that stuck with me the most was Sharon
Wachsler's "Still Femme." . . . I know, to a certain extent,
what it's like to feel your body changing while your concep-
tion of yourself remains unaltered. . . . These are issues that I
have perhaps struggled with the most. When my body changes
and I am no longer able to do things independently that I
once could, resentment swells. I can feel the mind–body relationship growing tense and frustrated. It feels out of control.
Being powerless over your own body is terrifying. (Amy)*

Our next session addresses "Disability as Difference, Identifying as a Disabled Woman, and Assistance and Self-definition."
Our readings include an account by an eighty-year-old woman with
arthritis, an essay on chronic migraine headache, and an article by a
deaf woman with a deaf daughter. We discuss what is gained from
viewing a disability as a difference, as well as what is lost when the
difficulties, limitations, and invisible work required to become able
are overlooked.

This week we begin to notice the degree to which women are
reluctant to identify as disabled. The students find—in their first
interviews with disabled women and in their own self-reflections—
that the word "disability" carries much negative weight. Someone
else seems always to be the disabled one, someone with a more
severe condition. The stigma associated with disabilities is underlying, I think, the sense that a disability is something a person would
rather not have because it makes them feel less valuable or capable.

*One thing Jodi said that stood out to me was "I'm not sure if I
am what you are looking for." . . . It seems as if she was unsure
if her invisible disabilities counted as disabilities. . . . We discussed the term disability after I asked if she was comfortable
identifying herself as disabled. She told me that "disabled" is*

an umbrella term and that it is not descriptive enough, for she certainly does not believe that her condition is the same as a physical disability. She considers her disability to define a large part of her being, but is very optimistic in telling me "it is not something I'll be stuck with forever." I was really glad for her. But should I be glad? I think that the reason I feel this way is because I am stuck in the mindset that disabilities all have a cure. (Joanna)

There is a moment Terry Galloway describes in her piece "I'm Listening As Hard As I Can" that I think almost every person with a disability has at least once in her life. . . . It is a moment when she can no longer maintain the façades that she has dubbed herself into believing: the idea that if you will it away hard enough, your disability will disappear, if you ignore it then it doesn't exist. I have felt that because my disability makes me physically weaker, I had to be mentally stronger. The way I could outsmart my disability was to show no sign that it affected me, negatively or positively. I would take on everything a person without a disability did and then more. I had to do more, always. I felt that I had to somehow make up for my disability by excelling in every aspect my disability didn't affect. (Amy)

Our readings in this and future weeks suggest that an identification as disabled is something women often come to later in life. Georgina Kleege talks about her blindness being the same when she was eleven years old as when she wrote her book, *Sight Unseen*: "Writing this book made me blind," she notes. Mairs discusses how her disability becomes part of her self-identity that she cannot imagine herself without. In our other accounts, the different sensibility and culture that having a disability creates is suggested in readings on both blindness and deafness. The issue of personal assistance appears in an article on ethical dilemmas of sign language interpreters, who must consider to whom they owe their allegiance—the deaf persons they are interpreting for, the hearing people listening, or their own sense of appropriateness.

> *Of the blindness and vision readings, I particularly liked Alexander's description of when she visited a school for the deaf, and she asked the children if they ever received the question "would you rather be blind or deaf?" I think that her observation, that answering with the disability that you have, is a way of accepting your situation and adjustment to your lifestyle. I also think that it makes perfect sense that you would grow accustomed to the senses you do have and in turn not be able to imagine life without the sense that you have grown to rely on. (Sylvia)*

In class discussion, the students now ask me, "What qualifies as a disability?" They are concerned about conducting their interviews with disabled women and feel it is about time we defined our subject. They will be interviewing a disabled woman for an hour and a half each week during the next three weeks, and then later in the course, pursuing a topic that interests them. This series of conversations with disabled women at first seems daunting to the students. "How will I find disabled women?" they ask, feeling they don't know any. They soon become aware of the presence of disabled women all around them. I tell them that they can define disability in any way that feels right to them, their definitions can change over time, and that giving a few examples to others they interview often helps. We go around the seminar table sharing our definitions. As I offer mine, I am surprised to find how much it hinges on self-worth. "Anything that makes me feel devalued limits what I feel I can do," I say. "It disables me." The students' definitions tend to emphasize that a disability puts a woman in a minority, that it may be viewed negatively by the outside world but is essentially a difference, and that it may be positive for the individual, and they note that it depends on culture.

> *One definition of disability I still have is some difference in the person whether from a disease or an accident that makes them different from the normal in their society. Another . . . is a difference that affects the body and mind and from those effects it has brought about hardships. (Mary Beth)*

The students describe their interviews in their papers each week and share them in class, offering them outward like a series of mini-dramas. In the interview assignments I give, I ask them to note and reflect on how they each feel at the time of the interview, rather than simply writing about what the other woman says. I tell them that I think their responses and inner questions can help guide their learning and provide them with a sense of grounding, which I have found in my own research experiences. Their self-reflections also make their papers more interesting for me to read, because I then feel more in touch with each student.

> *Before the interview, . . . I expected myself to have awkward thoughts about my personal relationship with Rachel. . . . During the interview, I didn't think about any of that at all. I was engaged with what she was saying and learning about her experiences of diabetes. (Kathryn)*

> *My interview was of a fellow graduate student, Chris, who has bi-polar disorder and fibromyalgia. . . . I was specifically interested in her experiences with invisible disabilities and how her disabilities affect her as a mother. . . . When I listened to the*

interview on my computer, I thought about how I felt. . . . This
interview gave me a tangible experience with someone who is
very similar to the speakers in the readings. (Sara)

I interviewed one of my friends who is hard-of-hearing or
legally deaf. . . . I went to high school with Kimberly and
due to that closeness, I could slightly push her further than
I would be able to a stranger. First thing I did was ask her
if she viewed herself as disabled and she immediately was
like "noooo." I said, "Then tell me what you view as disabled"
while thinking, "I can see how she doesn't view herself as dis-
abled but at the same time, I had doubt." (Mary Beth)

In week four, our subject is "Invisible Realities: Emotional
Disabilities." The first year I taught the course, I included only one
reading on emotional disabilities, Mairs's "On Living Behind Bars."
I did not devote extended attention to the topic. Then one year a
graduate student who had dealt with serious depression gave us a
reading she liked and encouraged further exploration. I found that
the students were highly interested. Often they had had depressive
periods themselves and knew other women students with emotional
disabilities whom they wished to understand. I therefore sought to
expand my repertoire, now devoting a full week. Our main reading
is Kay Redfield Jamison's *An Unquiet Mind* on manic depression—a
book I felt lucky to find because Jamison speaks of mental illness in
such a clear way that the sense of chaos and underlying dark threat
and abyss—that I, at least, have always associated with mental illness—is made to seem understandable. Jamison recommends both
medication and psychotherapy in a way I find fair-minded. We have
several other readings and are able to have an intelligent discussion of emotional disabilities that previously I was not sure I could
achieve. Our emotional disabilities discussion helps the students to

think about emotional dimensions of all the disabilities we consider during the rest of the term.

The students usually look forward to our emotional disabilities week and are grateful for our discussion. However, I approach this week with trepidation, for I know I will want to tell them about my own experiences. From the start of the quarter, I have told the students about my blindness, using it to provide a personal example of looking at a disability of one's own and drawing insights from it. But my emotional difficulties are much harder for me to discuss. My initial hesitance about including emotional disabilities in the course was, I think, because this subject felt too close to home for me. I have had profound emotional difficulties all my life—such as destructive, self-critical inner voices that can incapacitate me by undermining my sense of self-worth and ability to act; extreme anxiety when speaking with people for fear that I will be found unacceptable; and a deep lack of trust in my ability to be safe. Yet I tend to keep such troubles private for fear of rejection or misunderstanding. I feel that my emotional challenges separate me from others whose lives seem easier to manage. In my mind, emotional disabilities are the most stigmatized, particularly my own.

When I teach my course, I must overcome the very fears that characterize my difficulties. I face a dilemma: although I want to speak of my emotional troubles, I fear that the students will pull away from me if they know I have them. Will they feel that I am not stable enough to be their teacher, not want to learn from me, or expect that I will become too needful? At the same time, I know that if I am silent I will be contributing to the further stigmatization of emotional illness and the shame surrounding it. To solve my dilemma, I have developed a strategy of telling the students, first, that it is harder for me to speak of my emotional disability than of my blindness, and then that I have learned some things from my blindness that have helped me with my emotional difficulties and vice versa.

With my blindness, I explain, it has been obvious to me from the start that I must do much extra hidden work to compensate or manage. I have had to learn to do things differently, take extra steps, feel with my hands for objects that someone else might see, use aids like a guide dog or a white cane to be safe, learn new computer skills, and, most of all, I have had to learn not to expect to see. On the contrary, with my emotional disability, I have tended to expect— perhaps because my emotional difficulties are so invisible and easily denied—that I should not have them, and that I should not have to do extra work to deal with them. I have expected that my emotional troubles will magically get better, and I have viewed myself as a failure when they do not—when my emotions get me down.

I tell the students that I have learned from my blindness that I must confront my emotional troubles with a more open spirit. I must say to myself, "Now this—the emotional difficulty—takes extra work, just like your lack of sight. You must stop, go outside, do something that will make you feel better. Don't be so hard on yourself. Talk to yourself. Talk it down. Talk back to the inner destructive voices. Tell someone else about it. It's not going to magically go away. It's an extra job. It comes with the territory. Take care of something. You will feel you are taking care of yourself." Such inner conversation is not new to me, but viewing my emotional difficulties as a disability is. To me, that means that my emotions require extra work. They require that I take a kind of inner time out—to recover and rebuild—that I recognize the legitimacy of my emotional troubles, the givenness of them, and that alleviating steps are necessary. These steps include asking for help from others.

Viewing my emotional troubles as a disability is something I did not do before teaching Women and Disabilities, but I find that it makes these troubles seem more tangible and coherent to me and less like a personal failure. It also explains why I have always felt that I was "working all the time" with respect to my emotions in order to feel safe. My inner work, in the past, has felt like a burden to me and like no one else had to do it. But viewing this work as what comes with a disability makes it feel more natural and acceptable.

In the reverse, I tell the students, my having had to deal with emotional difficulties for a long time has prepared me for my blindness, which has always seemed easier for me to deal with. I think this is because my blindness is more external, more socially recognized as a disability, and not viewed as my fault—as a result of a lack of a willingness to do better. My blindness does not feel as potentially life-threatening or internally painful as my inner thoughts can be. Yet my emotional disability has marked me for so long that I cannot imagine myself without it, nor do I want to be without it. My emotional life, although difficult at times, is also the rich inner life that grounds me. It has taught me that, in confronting any other disability, such as my blindness, I must always look inside myself for possible negative internalizations and effects on my self-esteem. The outer physical disability is never the crucial problem, which is, rather, the effects on the inner self.

When I speak to the students about my emotional disability in comparison with my blindness, I hope they will understand. Although I am nervous, my words come out more clearly than I ever expected; the time goes by quickly. I can hear the students listening with respectful attention, and then we move on.

This week for my self-reflective research, I went on two 30 minute walks alone to just think and clear my head. After the second walk, I laid in bed, eyes closed, and just tried to start from the beginning. . . . The disability I chose to write about was my bipolar type 2 disorder. . . . Before last year, I never really felt anything about my disorder because I didn't really have one in my eyes. I just thought I was a moody teenage girl. I was someone who was surrounded by great friends and family but felt so alone. . . . [Last year,] I was forced to take a medical leave and admitted to the hospital for severe depression where the doctors diagnosed me as bipolar. . . . It was so weird to have a name to it. I, at the time, was uneducated about mental illnesses so I only had this idea about bipolar from what the media had concocted. As the doctor began to explain everything to me, it became more clear to me. All those times I thought I was just an overly emotional woman, I wasn't. I just had something different in me. (Mary Beth)

One insight that was meaningful to me comes from Jamison's psychiatrist's notes when he recorded, "Patient reluctant to be with people when depressed because she feels her depression is such an intolerable burden on others." When I feel depressed, I feel the same way. I am critical, sarcastic and negative. Sometimes I will try to be positive and hope that being around others will pull me up or at least put pressure on me to psych myself into a good mood. But in the end it is too hard to please-excuse-yourself-from-the-table because you've had a sudden sink in mood, without causing a lot of fuss. . . . Is it true that people don't really want to be around depressed persons, or is that a signature feeling of depression that I only understand because I have been depressed? For me this raises a big issue I have with any psychological disorder: given your mind is the only one you know, how are you supposed to recognize when it is normal or not? (Kathryn)

Our topics in week five are "Ideas of Beauty and of Female Acceptability, Passing and Invisible Work, and Caretaking and Self-care." We read Lorna Moorhead's *Coffee in the Cereal*, a lively book about her first year with multiple sclerosis that details her efforts to pass as nondisabled by keeping up a conventional female cosmetic appearance. She wears high heels although she totters when walking and must constantly grasp objects to steady herself. She puts on makeup so she will "look nice," although then other people, including doctors, do not believe she is very sick or needs help. Moorhead calls her efforts "compensating for lost parts," describing how initially she was surprised by the degree to which her compensating exhausted her. Her desires not to appear defective, ungraceful, ugly, less beautiful than she might be, less desirable as a woman, are echoed by quite a few of our other authors. Accompanying a concern with appearance in their accounts is a parallel concern with maintaining accustomed female caretaking habits. Nancy Mairs and Sharon Wachsler, for example, describe how when they can no longer do the physical caretaking of others they once did, they try in other ways, such as in speaking with people and giving advice, or in accepting help from others so that they will not cause others to worry about them.

The students readily identify with the female beauty concerns raised in this week's readings. They often surprise me with their acceptance of the necessity for makeup and for very stereotypically female dress styles. I sit in the classroom feeling I am so much less conventional than they are, but I know that, as I became increasingly blind, I began worrying more about my clothes matching and not looking unkempt, and about whether I would be able to continue to care for others—my intimate partner, my animals and plants—betraying, I think, my own version of clinging to conventional female gender roles. These roles often feel to me like a protection against losing a sense of value, a guarding of my personal acceptability; my female gender seems so obviously tied to my sense of safety, the roles all the more needed because of the vulnerabilities I feel as a result of my disabilities.

The topics Moorhead focused on are very female, such as make-up, high-heels and motherhood. The way in which she discusses her conflict with attention and how people perceive

*her is also particularly feminine. In overcoming daily chal-
lenges, she wants people to acknowledge both how hard she
works to live with a disability and the independence she currently has, which is often impossible, leaving her with little
satisfaction. This apparent need for validation comes up over
and over again in my interviews with college women with
disabilities. (Joanna)*

*Like in most of the stories we read this week, my illness [has]
also affected my physical being which I attributed so much
to my femininity. With makeup, I can be beautiful. With
clothes, I can look thin. But with illness, I am not beautiful
in my eyes or anyone else's. Why does this shift occur and how
can we as a society portray beauty in all shapes, sizes, and
disabilities? (Mary Beth)*

This past year, I included in our "Ideas of Beauty" week two
accounts of autism that further develop themes of caretaking and
female behavioral appropriateness, in addition to emphasizing how different it is to be in an autistic sensory world. Eileen Garvin's *How to Be
a Sister* describes her relationship with her autistic adult sister, providing a reminder of how often women become the caretakers of the disabled. She notes that in families, it is almost always the sisters of autistic
siblings who assume they will have a lifetime caretaking responsibility.
One student in class this year related especially to the account:

*How to Be a Sister provides so many insights that I could
relate to! Because I grew up with a younger brother who has
autism. . . . Right now, I feel that my brother's life is not his
own. We are constantly in a struggle to make him behave normally. Even though he is becoming more independent as he
grows up, I still believe that he will need to be taken care of*

forever. I expect that once my parents are gone, I will be the one to take him into my home. From reading this book, I've learned that this doesn't have to be the case. There are options. (Joanna)

In week six, our focus turns to "Autoimmune Diseases among Women: Prevalence, Attitudes, and Themes." Among our readings are several on chronic fatigue and immune dysfunction syndrome (CFIDS) that describe personal experiences of women in medical situations where their complexity of symptoms with invisible and unknown cause is not taken seriously. Susan Cahn shows how the lack of external recognition can cause extreme self-doubt and inner confusion. She reflects on the constant challenge of explaining herself to others and on the importance of respecting her own sense of her illness. Susan Wendell articulates a common dilemma—that because at times she seems healthy, people expect her to be more able than she is. They do not realize how much she must parcel out her time and effort because her periods of severe fatigue will return. Similarly, in her article on lupus, "Spoon Theory," Christine Miserandino describes her daily life in terms of being allotted a set of spoons. Each effort to do something takes a spoon. She must plan her activities for the day carefully to do what she wants. When the spoons are gone, she can do no more. She is acutely conscious of her calculations, but she knows others are not.

In their assignment for this week, I ask the students to speak briefly with a variety of women, rather than conducting one interview. Their assignment is to ask at least five women about other women they know who have autoimmune diseases, and to note the language they use, the attitudes, prejudices, and assumptions toward the disabled women. The students are impressed with the range of autoimmune conditions they uncover and that our readings suggest—allergies, Crohn's disease, thyroid disease, multiple sclerosis, asthma, rheumatoid arthritis, CFIDS, scleroderma. They share their reports from the field:

During my first interview, I somehow (wrongly) assumed that even if I did not know what an autoimmune disease was, that the people I interviewed would. . . . [When Jennifer didn't,] we decided to pull up the Wikipedia page, and it was there that she was able to look at the list and realize that she in fact knew of three women with an autoimmune disease. (Sylvia)

The first girl I talked to was Patricia who said that she had a family friend that has MS and is in her thirties. . . . I noticed that Patricia did not know very much about the disease and spoke about it in a distant way. . . . She noted, that no one ever mentions the disease at gatherings when the woman is present. She emphasized that the situation is "so sad" and that the woman is "going to die young." . . . She says that the woman has a "strong personality" that has gotten sharper with the intensity of the disease. She said this without judgment, but I found it interesting that she attributed the woman's temper to the pain. From the class readings, I can deduce that this woman's impatience may be because of other frustrations of social misunderstanding. (Sara)

Although the students are discussing the lives of others, they are involving themselves as well:

I had a very strong response to the Goranson reading [on chronic fatigue syndrome], as her case seemed to be one of the more severe. My heart sank as she described how her once very full life had been reduced to perhaps leaving the house once a day to go to the post office, if she was feeling up to the challenge. An idea that she brought up was very similar to one that I think Mairs did in a reading from a previous week—that of no longer being able to identify yourself through actions. "Today, what a person does tends to define who a person is." . . . The suddenness of her symptom onset really affected me. The reading itself made me feel claustrophobic, and I literally had to get up and go do something after I finished the article, after I read how she was confined to her couch for so long. (Sylvia)

I could feel the complex and still not fully processed thoughts Christine Miserandino had towards Lupus. How it is something that makes you look at your life in a highly calculated manner but in a subconscious way. It becomes innate and a part of the way you live your life that you forget other people don't do this too. . . . The part that spoke to me the most is when Christine talks about learning to keep pace with her Lupus, which is usually a slower pace than she wants. (Amy)

I include in week six an account of breast cancer and two about sudden injury from automobile accidents that reveal processes of coming to terms with unexpected disability. These readings contain parallel themes to those found in the autoimmune accounts and highlight the inner resolve of the authors. Although the students are not aware of it, I am very conscious of the fact that I am now including breast cancer among the readings for the course, where initially I was afraid to include it. My sister had breast cancer not long ago, and it has always been a lurking specter for me simply because I am a woman. Again, as with my emotional difficulties, I feel an uneasiness when a disability approaches mine, but I know I must overcome my fears to include it.

The students, too, show that they are not withdrawing but, rather, becoming more immersed and more capable of reflecting on disabilities of their own. Each week when they write of their disability experiences, they take me with them in their daily life activities, revealing more aspects of their experiences, looking for themes also brought up in our readings, and further exploring their research topic. I always feel privileged to be reading their self-reflective accounts:

> *For self-reflective research this week, I took my bike to Trader Joe's for a food shopping trip. . . . This shopping trip was different [than usual] because I was self-reflective about why I picked the foods I did. . . . I wrote [a diary entry that night] and read for about forty-five minutes. I also read old e-mails from a particularly loving friend who knows my whole story. . . . My disability is that I still carry remnants of an eating disorder I had in the beginning of college. This was four years ago for me. My disability is inherently female because I now believe that it stemmed from repression of my emotional and sexual desires which I channeled into my physical appetite. (Sara)*

> *In my self reflection, I thought about how I try not to burden people with unnecessary information, and how that is a very female thing to do. One of the authors discusses how it took her such a long time to accept her CFIDS, and when she finally did, it took her several more years to tell her friends and family what that diagnosis actually entailed. A part of it I think was that she didn't want to be a burden, but I also think she didn't want them to see the way in which it changed her. This is an emotion I can highly relate to. When I was having my gallbladder problems, I know that I didn't want to burden the people around me with detail, and I also didn't want to be viewed as the "sick girl." . . . Nor did I want to be viewed as a complainer. So if people did something wrong, or didn't treat me in a way that I expected, I would just put it in the back of my mind, and try and move on. . . . However over time these small slights build, and rarely, but sometimes, . . . I will just simply get fed up and*

let the person who has slighted me know everything that they have done, all at once. I think the main point to gain from the readings, interviews, and self reflection this week is that it is important to have open communication between women with disabilities and the people they engage with in order to ensure that everyone's emotional needs are being met. (Sylvia)

The students' self-reflections often show a desire to avoid the appearance of weakness that may be associated with femaleness:

For my self-reflective research this week, I returned to the topic of menstrual cramps. . . . Having my period and everything that comes with it is always a secret. When my cramps prevent me from attending class, I would email my teacher telling him/ her that I am sick. If I get cramps during work, I tell my boss I need to go home because of a headache. I feel that telling them the truth would make me seem weak, embarrassed, incapable. Even my feminine hygiene products are hidden—I always keep them in the most obscure pockets of my bags. In my room, I never put them out in the open. When I take medicine for my pains, I also do it quickly and privately. . . . I don't want to make my period visible because that would make my female-ness visible. We live in a culture where periods and PMS are depicted so often as excuses for weakness. . . . Because of painful periods, I give up hours, sometimes days, of productivity in school work. I put in much more hidden work than just once a month. I must schedule my activities and travel around the possibility of getting a period. I keep a notecard of emergency contacts in my purse, mostly so that I can call someone to come save me in case my cramps cause me to black out or not make it home. . . . Periods, especially painful ones, feel like such a disability to me. (Joanna)

When we next turn to "Disability as Adventure; Personal Identity; and Alternate Ways of Seeing," the students read my book, *Traveling Blind: Adventures in Vision with a Guide Dog by My Side*, a narrative about my coming to terms with my blindness as I travel with Teela as a new guide dog, exploring my surroundings with changed sight. The students like the personal style of *Traveling Blind* and feel it helps equalize our sharing, since they have been writing to me about their personal disability experiences and their subjective responses to our readings for some time now in their weekly papers. I notice that after reading my writing, the students speak more freely and honestly in their papers than they had before. I sometimes feel I find my voice in theirs—I will note similarities in our word use and vernacular writing style—and this will surprise me and, at the same time, please me. I think that the pleasure and recognition may go both ways. I cannot imagine teaching this course the way I do without having pieces of my own writing to share with the students, but I think a course such as this can be taught very personally even without first-person accounts on the part of the teacher. The important thing is encouraging the students' candid self-expression. Their papers on *Traveling Blind* express a generosity toward me for which I am grateful:

> *Your book taught me not to take any experience for granted or to dwell on the negatives whether you believe they are negative or society has told you it is negative. Dwelling on these things causes one to miss out on the great joy that is right in front of them and to forget that there are so many ways of experiencing the world. My favorite insight I came to realize when reading your book was holding on to my self-worth and self-confidence and never letting anyone define my identity or ultimately, myself. (Mary Beth)*

> *In the introduction, when you wrote that most people view vision as a binary, and assume you are either totally blind or*

seeing, I recognized that that is how I viewed vision as well before I began this course. (Sylvia)

I enjoyed reading the chapters "Are You Training That Dog?" and "Airport Stories" because I could sense so much of Susan's character as she finds her voice and public/private self. It is unfortunate that she had to face so many obstacles in order to define herself for public perception, but I find her stories very inspiring. I felt like I was with her along the way, feeling her self-judgment and self-consciousness. But I also celebrated with her as she began to speak up and ask for help. (Joanna)

The students' responses to *Traveling Blind* impress me with how nicely they mix their stories and inner perceptions with mine. They are both identifying with me through similarities we share and articulating their differences, while noting overall themes. These are skills they have been developing all along during the quarter:

The theme that stood out to me in Part 3 was hidden work. The amount of work and thought that Susan puts into her daily activities surprises me because they are things that I never have to consider, like being careful of the cat while cutting food on the kitchen counter. In addition to being worried about her actions, she is constantly preoccupied by the state of her sight. . . . In some ways, I feel that it must be tough being her. In other ways, I feel that my experiences aren't that different from hers, in that I face obstacles and adventures every day too, just in different ways. (Joanna)

In the second part I loved Chapter Six where the reader got to hear more about your childhood and understand what your family is like, if only for a small portion of the book. I liked

the associations that were drawn between Judaism and dis-
abilities. As a Jew with a disability, I think the eras are very
different. I have rarely felt discriminated against but I can
see how growing up in a time of war and persecution would
leave its mark for life. . . . [Later] I especially could relate to
Part Three with the airport stories and people asking about
the service dog. When I had my service dog, Victor, from sev-
enth to freshman year of college, people would always be com-
ing up to me to ask about him and tell me about their dog. I
didn't mind too much since I got to meet a lot of great people I
wouldn't have otherwise, but it did get a bit grating at times.
When I was younger, however, I loved that people were star-
ing at Victor and not me and my wheelchair. (Amy)

In our class discussion, the students often mention the positive outlook conveyed in *Traveling Blind*, since many of the chapters stress my sense of satisfaction, gratitude, and of appreciating
the world I now move in, and the book, in the end, emphasizes
self-acceptance. Previously in the quarter, the students have mentioned that they are finding a bias toward a positive outlook in our
readings for the course generally. The authors I have chosen often
achieve an equilibrium in relation to their disability, and often the
accounts have a positive tone in the ending, rather than being stories
of a descent into worse and worse misery. Joan Didion, for example,
ends her essay on migraine noting that her time of intense pain has
passed: "I notice a flower on the stairwell . . . I count my blessings."

I tell the students that, indeed, there may be a bias in my choice of
readings, and that there is also probably a bias in what gets published,
since publishers and editors will tend to select uplifting accounts. But
their comments suggest to me something more. I think that women
perhaps often do emphasize the positive—the gains, the comforting thoughts, a way of responding to and coming to terms with a

disability that is reassuring. Women often develop an inner outlook that is an antidote to the difficulties of a disability. Their accounts are often characterized by a drive toward self-acceptance and by an internal humor, typically at the expense of the self—something that lightens the weightiness of the disability. At least, that has been so in my own case. The picture I present in *Traveling Blind* is complete with difficulties, but these are not the emphasis—because my writing is one of the ways I try to make my disability better. Through the writing, I can convert the negatives to a positive, developing insights that help me to feel more comfortable with my blindness.

> *We had a good dinner that night back up in Silver City and I slept well. . . . But my dreams were back in that sunlit place where I had stood with my binoculars and looked up at a mountain and felt satisfied and happy. That moment was part of a longer day, a longer journey. . . . I wanted to remember and hold close some lessons I had learned that day from my travels. Though I had tried to see with acuity the changing landscape around me, more important to me were my moments of acceptance—when I saw without binoculars or telephoto lens; when I relished the ghostlike, the fuzzy town, the cactus with invisible spikes, the smell of cooking grease, the excitement of being in a borderland, the fur of my guide dog, the love I felt from Hannah. (Krieger, in* Traveling Blind*)*

In this week's assignment, I supplement the students' reading of *Traveling Blind* by asking them to listen to several public presentations I have given—on radio, television, and in a civic club—so they can get a sense of broader responses to the book. This year, for the first time, I gave them a copy of the new audiobook version of *Traveling Blind* so they could sample it and compare reading by listening—as a blind person does—with reading a text visually. I also gave them the text as a digital file so they could experiment with using the synthesized text-to-speech voices in their computers or phones reading the text aloud to them.

It took extra assertiveness on my part to ask the students to read samples of the book by listening—because I tend to keep hidden the alternative format work I do in reading and writing, not wanting to show that things take me more time. I also did not want to overload the students. However, they were grateful for the exposure to assistive technology. With regard to listening, they much preferred reading with their eyes and did not quite understand the purpose of the fairly flat reading cadence that I chose for the audiobook narration. That cadence, to me, closely approximates how I hear my writing. I pointed out to them that there is no expression on the visual printed page; all that is created in the reader's mind. As I did so, I became aware of how much it takes learning new skills to read through listening when blind, and that I have mastered and become accustomed to these skills more than I know.

> *Listening to the book on audio made me feel like I was seeing the action, as if I were watching a movie with my eyes closed. I was better able to imagine movements, physical interactions, and the visual environment. When I read Chapter 5 in print, it was very difficult for me to keep track of the author's movement and location. The audio allowed me to better imagine where she was going. . . . I feel that the print allowed me to better sense emotions. (Joanna)*

> *I prefer reading in print, because I can move at my own pace, and give my own inflection. I felt that the story was more exciting when I could put my own inflection in the voice. If I had to rely on another person's voice to read all my materials, . . . I can imagine that I would start to feel affection for*

the voice and think of it as a friend. Like all friends; how-
ever, you need more than six hours with them before you start
trusting them. (Sara)

When I first opened the VoiceOver program I thought wow,
this technology is really cool and fun! But very quickly I turned
from thinking it was fun to a pain in the ass. I wanted to rush
through the tutorial program because all I wanted to know
was how to hear the text in a word document, not [learn how
to] navigate my computer with the VoiceOver commands. . . .
Eventually the VoiceOver program began to read through the
text continuously, but still with annoying pauses at the end of
each line. I think if I were not entering this experience as an
assignment I may have been able to slow down and enjoy the
technology more; as it was, I was overwhelmed with frustra-
tion! (Kathryn)

The students' responses to the public presentations showed the
influence of their learning in the course:

When I heard some of the excerpts read to the Commonwealth
Club, I felt that they were taken more humorously than when
I read them. The audience giggled when they heard about you
finding a place for Teela to pee in the airport, but when I read
that portion of the book I read it with a more serious tone.
When I watched you on the video segment, . . . I liked how
you answered the interviewer's question about fear [of your
blindness] and summarized how the book took that fear and
turned it into something positive: an adventure. (Kathryn)

In your Commonwealth Club presentation and YouTube pro-
gram, you presented your work with such poise and presence that

was in direct reaction to the stereotype of people with blindness and even broader, with disabilities, as inept. When you said because you move slowly, you fear people will think of you as dumb, a light bulb went off in my head. This world, especially America, is such a fast-paced country both literally and figuratively that society places this negative stigma on those who do not keep up with them as people with less worth. This negativity is then rubbed off onto the person with the disability. (Mary Beth)

During Susan's presentation, I really liked her insight on her experience being an outsider. Because she was used to feeling like an outsider in being a woman, lesbian, and Jewish, losing sight did not feel like a completely new experience. I could really relate to her statement because I often feel like an outsider too, being female, Asian, and Buddhist. I felt really glad when she said that offers of help and condescension could be good. This was reassuring to me because I am often afraid to interact with disabled people, even through offering help, because I fear coming off as offensive. (Joanna)

As we discuss *Traveling Blind*, I am particularly aware of Teela's comforting presence as she lies under the seminar table at my feet, an invisible but intrinsic part of the educational process. It is no coincidence that the title of my book, and of this week's topic in the course, has the word "adventure" in it. For I doubt that I would have used that term, or thought of my blindness in such a positive manner, had I not had her in my life. In the classroom, when we discuss *Traveling Blind*, the students ask me about how I got her and further questions concerning guide dogs, linking this to issues of assistive technology more broadly. I ask them not to refer to Teela by name in our discussion, but to call her "Big Dog" as we do at home, or something similar, so that she does not immediately get up and ask if I want her to take me somewhere. In discussing my blindness and my emotional life with the students, I feel more comfortable being honest with them because I have Teela with me. I feel she makes me seem more accessible to them, and that her presence helps all of us feel "at home" in the classroom—more willing to share.

In week eight, our topics are "Intimate Relationships, Complex Emotionality, and Personal Assistance and Self-determination." We read Beth Finke's *Long Time, No See*, a book about her "two companions"—diabetes and blindness as a result of her diabetes. I like Finke's account because it is extremely honest and multifaceted. The students like it and are engrossed but are also concerned because Finke does not live up to certain ideals they have about how a disabled woman should be. For instance, she describes her initial rejecting emotions upon giving birth to a severely disabled child and discusses confronting her husband's infidelity, possibly related to her way of dealing with her disability. As I listen to the students speak in class about their responses to the book, I am dismayed that they do not appreciate it exactly as I do, that they are often negatively judgmental of the author. At the same time, I hope that exposing them to the account will make them more accepting of unexpected inner realities of others in the future, and more accepting of such complexities within themselves.

I loved the [chapter] title of "My Two Companions" because when a disease or a disorder have been with you for so long; they do become your companion. I used to say that I couldn't go out because depression wants me to stay in. I would not particularly call my bipolar a companion because companion has a more positive connotation than I would attribute to the majority of my episodes but I understand where she is coming from. When everybody and everything has abandoned you, your disability or disease will always be there. (Mary Beth)

It was difficult for me to read Finke without continually feeling bad for her. I found myself asking, "How can so many unfortunate things happen to one person?" I know that we are taught in this class to view disability as difference, but I couldn't help feeling that the experiences Finke went through were all unfortunate and bad. . . . It was both frustrating and encouraging to know that she carried a very positive attitude throughout. Frustrating because I couldn't understand why she wasn't as angry as I expected; encouraging because she led life with such a strong sense of self-determination and resilience. (Joanna)

We further consider the issue of self-determination in discussing two articles on personal assistance and abuse by Mary Frances Platt, who presents a list of guidelines for assisting a disabled woman that emphasize doing what the disabled woman wants, even if it is not your way, for example, of caring for a pet. When we discuss these articles, I always think back to the initial year of the course when I was preparing my first syllabus. I asked a disabled student whose opinion I valued what she would suggest I be sure to include that I might overlook. "Personal assistance," she said immediately. She had been disabled from birth, used a wheelchair, and needed always to employ assistants. She then told me, "You know, most of the students who take the course are going to be premeds." She knew far more than I did at that time. I am also reminded of a year when a student then taking the course, disabled and in a wheelchair from an auto accident, described for the class how important to her sense of identity small items could be. "I like to wear overalls," she said. "But my assistant feels I should wear elastic waist pants instead, because they are easier to get on and off. I feel there is no question, that even if it is harder, the way I dress is an expression of my identity. So I am wearing overalls today."

I was strongly moved by her statement since I feel similarly, reacting against limitations imposed by others when they are not mine. Students in my class and others often feel that decisions should be mutual between a disabled woman and her assistant, while I always feel the disabled woman should have the final say, so I find it useful to remember back to that student with her overalls asserting her identity.

> *Lastly, do not ignore someone's disability but at the same time, do not pity or think you are better. Acknowledge the disability and ask what you can do to assist them, not help but assist. Helping seems to say that I am giving you my greater abilities because I am better off while assisting is simply just what the word signifies, assisting the individual to reach their own goal. (Mary Beth)*

> *It is absolutely an unexpected social drain when the care-giving relationship is not what both parties desire. . . . I have become the emotional support of many care-givers as their lives come crumbling down and all they have left is their job, working with me. It is impossible for their outside life to not affect their performance, or at least their personality, at work. This often places me in an awkward position because while I am willing to be supportive, I am also their employer. I have had to fire care-givers because they have brought so much stress and negativity into the workplace that it significantly affects me for the worse. (Amy)*

The theme of "Breaking Silences, Claiming Identity, and Seeking Community" makes great sense for the next-to-last week of the term. Several of our readings in week nine describe how the authors did not identify as disabled until becoming involved with other disabled people and participating in a disabled rights movement. Mary Felstiner, with arthritis for many years, tells a story of first identifying as disabled when joining a demonstration. Other authors convey their sense of elation upon discovering a disabilities community and describe how they then reconsidered themselves, reviewing their pasts, and asking why they had not identified as disabled before. Some accounts are highly individual. Judith Moses, for example, describes a personal journey of coming to accept that she had a disability she had never wanted to view as her own because her mother had it. These writings suggest a feeling of greater inner peacefulness when the author breaks her silences or acknowledges having a disability, if only to herself. They also suggest that such acknowledgment is often followed by a desire to help others who are disabled. Our readings this week further echo themes found earlier in the quarter, particularly concerning feelings of being different experienced by disabled women, the inner emotional struggles confronted, and the importance of how a woman views herself.

> *The reading I immediately connected with this week is Joan Tollifson's "Imperfection is a Beautiful Thing: On Disability and Meditation." She opens in the second paragraph her dream of a world where her disability is normal, where people don't try to make it into something other than what it means to the individual. This is something I strongly relate to. Sometimes I wonder what it would be like if I had grown up in a society where having a disability was not seen as different, either positive or negative. (Amy)*

This week the students submit one of two final papers—a final research process paper, for which they review their prior weekly papers, focusing on the interview and self-reflection sections. Here they have the opportunity to explore the development of their own narrative voices. I ask them to examine their learning process over time and to tell me, "What has happened to your voice in these papers? How has it changed? What has happened to your ideas and your topic? What themes concerning female gender seem most important to you now?" When I read their review papers, I am moved by how thoughtfully the students speak of changes in their written voices. The intimate narrative research and writing style that I have been encouraging seems rewarding to them, and they notice, as I did while reading their weekly papers throughout the quarter, that there are meaningful improvements in what they are able to express:

I think that my response papers have become more intimate as the quarter has progressed. . . . In the third paper, I think I started to open up, especially surrounding my responses to the readings and the feelings they invoked. I started giving more intimate details about my thoughts and responses, and was more honest about emotions that weren't always the most flattering. I was willing to admit more, and that in turn made the paper more accessible. (Sylvia)

I became proud of my voice over the course of this quarter. At the beginning, I didn't know very much about disabilities: my own disabilities, those of others, or my thoughts about them. My voice portrayed this uncertainty for it was nervous, frustrated, helpless, desperate, insecure, and lonely. The words I used in my first paper to describe my disability were all very negative. . . . Looking back, I am impressed at how introspective, aware, curious, self-conscious, knowledgeable and confident I have become. I am an authority on my own feelings. . . . In the end, my voice is calm and free, open to experiences and accepting of differences. My words and phrases seem relaxed to me compared to those in my first paper. I am pleased at how my voice has found its place. (Joanna)

In their review papers, I am always impressed with the insights the students have gained about disabilities, their interview adventures, and their ideas about gender. I appreciate especially how conscientiously they have considered disability and disability-like experiences of their own. I remember the first year I taught the course, one student ingeniously identified as her disability: "I have no sense of direction. Other people can get in a car and go somewhere. I always get lost." Since then, the disability experiences have included: "I have a mysterious scalp condition." "I have lupus." "I feel overly guilty." "I have knee pain. I have no cartilage, so I can't dance anymore. It makes be sad because I used to do competitive Irish dancing." "I had a concussion, so I forget things and I get headaches." "I have a learning disability. I have to be very organized. I plan everything. When I go to the store, I have to make a list or I won't be able to do it." "I have manic depression. I was in the hospital three times last year, but I'm doing better." "I have trouble breathing. I have to use an inhaler." "One of my eyes doesn't work." "I'm bipolar. I'm seeing a therapist." "I have no horizon. That makes it hard for me to carry my tray." "I have a deteriorative muscle disease. People always want to be my friend, but I haven't had a romantic relationship yet." "I have cerebral palsy." "I am anorexic. I have to be very careful about food." "I have trouble speaking in groups." "I had a limp for a while. I had a problem in one eye. I hope it's not MS."

Still, when I ask the students in their final research process paper to tell me, "How do you feel now about applying the word disabled to yourself?" some of them feel comfortable with it, but others do not. One student mentioned to me in our last class this past year, "You seemed disappointed when we didn't all identify. Were you, and if so, why?" I had to admit that I was disappointed, because I felt they all were disabled in some way, and that identifying helped disabled people generally in increasing numbers and understanding. However, in class I reassured the students that it was okay with me if they did not identify.

In my teaching I do not criticize their choices, but affirm them, feeling that each statement of how they feel represents a present sense that is to be respected. Although the students might not identify now, I thought that, in the future, they would be able to identify if needed— for instance, if suddenly it seemed useful to them to think about a personal illness, a difference, a difficulty or life challenge they faced as a disability. Or if viewing an experience of their own as a disability helped them also to understand someone else, the identification could be a source of strength. They might sometimes identify, sometimes not, but they now had that ability. They could draw from within themselves to understand other disabled people rather than looking from outside.

> *I think one of my main reasons to resist labeling myself as disabled is the judgment that would come with it. Even my PC defense that I might offend others by calling myself disabled is in a way a fear of judgment. I think that I am especially afraid of being judged about very personal matters, and it shows in my papers around the topic of depression. (Kathryn)*

> *Even though I would not consider myself disabled, I do not deny my condition as disabling. I often feel great relief after talking to others who have similar experiences or who care enough to learn about my condition. But talking to people also means that I am exposing my private self, causing me to feel vulnerable to their judgments. (Joanna)*

The students often find helpful the idea that a disability is a gift, although they may have mixed feelings:

> *Tollifson calls being disabled a deep wound/source of pain that is also a gift. . . . For me, I think of my disability of not having a normal relationship to food being a symptom*

of other "wounds," to use Tollifson's wording. I struggle with thinking of my disability as a gift, because to me, it is annoying. It is not scary like it used to be for sure, since it is at bay, but it is not something I like to identify with. (Sara)

Before this class, I believed that I viewed disability simply in the physical medical terms of no longer having the ability to do something, whether it be walk, see, talk, hear, etc. I had never thought of my bipolar disorder or ADD as a disability mainly because those words are rarely used to describe but rather disorder is used. But after the class discussion, the readings, and the self-reflections, my definition has greatly changed. . . . It is a gift, a tool for learning, part of identity, a creator of community, and a companion. (Mary Beth)

Our final week is simply titled "Conclusion: Themes and Issues in the Lives of Disabled Women." The students contribute readings for the last class and write a course summary paper reviewing their readings from the entire quarter and their classroom experiences. Within this summary paper, I ask them to answer: "If you had to tell a stranger, what were the three most important things you learned this quarter, what would they be?" I also ask them to tell me about what they feel are their main accomplishments. I tend to need several summary exercises at the end of the term because we have been juggling so many different elements all along—the readings, the interviews with others, and the students' self-reflections. I tell the students that they will each have their own ways of integrating what they have learned and that articulating that is more important than what I might summarize for them.

Three main points that I would make when describing the class to a stranger are that first, there is a lot of invisible work that goes along with being a woman with a disability. Many aspects of disability are hidden even if it is obvious that the disability is not, and I would say that the majority of disabilities are hidden from the perspective of someone who simply sees you in public. Another important thing is that when it comes to interacting with others who are disabled, it is important to ask when you have a question—don't assume. Don't assume they want to be able to do something for themselves, or that they can't do something on their own. No one will be offended if you are sincerely trying to ask if you can help them. Also, just because someone has a disability does not mean they have any less life satisfaction than someone who is not disabled. Disabled women are not inherently unhappy, and often when they are unhappy it has more to do with the way in which they are being treated. (Sylvia)

If I had to tell a stranger three things about this class, the first thing I would lead with would be that everyone has a disability. Every individual should walk in another's shoes or in this case apply another title or stigma to yourself. By doing this, people can see how it feels and what negative stigmas they may have about that group of individuals. Another thing I would talk about is the vast amount of disabilities and that the definition of disability far exceeds what society paints it to be. (Mary Beth)

I would tell a stranger or someone I knew that one of the most important things I learned is that there is no one experience of disability. As obvious as this may seem, everyone experiences disability differently. I learned that it is fun for me to relate personally to things and to think about why I relate the way that I do. . . . I have also learned from this class that because people experience things differently it is useful to talk with

*others and hear about their perspective, and that it is possible
to pinpoint a difference in the way you and another view the
world without creating distance between you. (Kathryn)*

In our last class session this year, one of the students suddenly
captured our attention by referring back to the question she remembered asking in our very first class, "How do I relate to a disabled
person without offending them?" "I feel more comfortable now,"
she said. "I think it's because of the interviews you made us do." It
had not been my intention that the interviews address the students'
concern about how to relate to a disabled person without causing
offense, but I could not have been more pleased.

*Through interviewing disabled women, I practiced what I
would consider active listening—instead of passively writing down what the women told me, I keenly questioned and
examined my own thoughts throughout. In a way, I was
listening to myself at the same time I was listening to these
women. Being this kind of listener encouraged me to break
the silence, both in terms of interaction with others and in
formulating my own thoughts. (Joanna)*

*I learned how worried able-bodied people are about offend-
ing or being insensitive to someone with a disability. . . . I
think this insight into how nerve-racking it is gives me more
of an impetus to start the conversation about my disability.
I should be the one taking the lead instead of waiting to see
if it is a topic the person wants to approach but doesn't know
how to. I am better able to address the concerns and guide the
person in telling them it's ok to be nervous and uncomfortable
because I am more than happy to talk through their questions,
even if they're worried it might be offensive. (Amy)*

I always feel sad when our last class is over, and gone with it that private world of discussing topics and sharing our personal experiences. Will the students go out into the larger society and see what I wished them to see? Will their insights stay with them? Will they use their learning to make a better world and to find strength within themselves? I feel my course contributes but a small drop in the bucket in increasing understandings of disabilities. I emphasize certain themes, but I overlook others. Perhaps most of all, I contribute a sense of pride—my pride in being a woman, in having a disability, in braving inner emotional difficulties. The students have braved their difficulties, as well, and shared their emotional lives with me, and they have felt accomplished in the end.

> *Four themes that I've identified from this course are as follows: 1) Women perform a large amount of hidden work in living with a disability, 2) Women consider appearance as a priority concern in passing as nondisabled, 3) Women often play the role of caretaker even with disability, and 4) Disability causes a loss of identity for women. In self-reflection of my own disability and interviewing others for views of their own disabilities, I've found these themes to be consistently present. I think that as a woman, I am especially hard on myself for proving my own independence, competence, and credibility. I feel that having a disability jeopardizes all of these characteristics. So in order to overcome this obstacle, I have to pay extra attention to control my hidden work, appearance, and caretaking roles in order to prove my capability and secure my identity. I don't want a disability to take away my identity so I work hard not to accept it, but to hide it. I think this coping mechanism exists because I'm a woman. (Joanna)*

After the last class session this past year, as I chatted outside with one of the students before she went on her way, I glanced down at Teela standing beside me in the late afternoon sun. As I reached down to pet her, I recalled how, the first year I taught the course, a blind student had arrived with a guide dog, a lively Golden Retriever who lay under the table at her feet. I had then only begun to use a white cane, but that was the beginning of my desire for a dog. Two years later, when I applied to guide dog training school, I asked for a Golden Retriever just like hers. Now my dog lies under the table, reminding me that, in more ways than I know, teaching my Women and Disabilities course has involved and changed me, as it has the students. When I began the course, I was concerned about what to exclude. Since then, I have expanded my repertoire to include more and more types of disabilities. I think that seeing disability as a common experience in everyone is not an approach unique to me, but reflects a very female tendency to see need, vulnerability, inter-dependence; to wish to take care; and to want to prompt mutual identification. As the quarter ends, I am grateful for the students' accomplishments and insights:

> *As a student in your class, I feel that I have learned so many relevant skills. . . . I've learned about disabilities through women's personal accounts, bringing to life a topic that is so hidden and taboo. I've learned to approach and talk to women with disabilities behind the guise of the interviews, something I've always wished I were more comfortable at doing but never had the opportunity to. I've learned how to write personally, honestly, and fearlessly, representing the truth without having to claim authority, generalize observations, or argue opinions on anything except for my own thoughts. Perhaps you could include these insights as well as other student reactions to taking this course. (Joanna)*

*The life of a woman is an emotional journey but even more
so for a disabled woman. Society is constantly telling me as
well as other disabled women that we are not normal, that
we are not capable of doing what they do, that we should
question our happiness because society seems to say that with
the loss of normalcy comes a loss of happiness. But I disagree.
I am choosing to break my silence about being stereotyped,
about not using the term "disabled," not being open about my
disability, or how I have let society label me and define me. I
am more than a stigma and I am claiming my identity, my
complete identity. I, Mary Beth Williams, am a 20-year-old
woman who has bipolar disorder. I am part black, Native
American, and Puerto Rican; I come from a single parent
household that is considered low-income. I am breaking my
silence. . . . By doing this, I am redefining to myself what
it means to be sane, what it means to be disabled, what it
means to be black, much like Alice Walker redefined beauty for
herself. My disability does not need society's pity or mourning
because my disability is a gift. A gift that has taught me to see
life in a way others cannot or are unable to and in this way,
they are actually the ones who are disabled. (Mary Beth)*

Teaching my Women and Disabilities course has been an emotional journey for me as well. When I began, the subject was new to me. I had just started to lose my eyesight and had yet to explore all that would entail. Each time I taught the course, I learned more about the subtleties of having a disability. I learned how to speak of myself with greater ease, how to accept myself with more confidence. I came to the class at first unaccompanied, then accompanied by a golden guide dog. I came with memories of prior years of teaching the class, yet each term was a new challenge for me, requiring that I extend myself as a teacher in the same way as I asked the students to extend themselves—to probe deeply within for ways of seeing that could aid in dealing with disabilities or with any meaningful challenge in life. Much that I have learned about how to see myself in the face of my blindness, my emotions, and my being different in the world has been refined and enhanced by the shared learning I have done with several generations of students in this intensive course. I wish to thank them for so enriching my life.

May–November 2011 and June 2014

FOURTEEN

+ ◆◆◆◆ +

A New Pair of Eyes

HIS NAME IS FRESCO. He arrived five months ago, a yellow Labrador Retriever eighteen months old, much like Teela in stature and deferential temperament, though slightly smaller and a very different dog. That difference has been hard for me to adjust to, since I keep wanting him to be her. I want him to look exactly like her, to feel her body under his skin. I want him to guide me in that jubilant way she does, and, most of all, I have wanted from the start for him to bring me a Frisbee. But Fresco, although a retriever by breed, is not a retriever deep in his blood in the same way as Teela. Retrieving is not his life, his first nature. His first nature is his desire for companionship, and second to that, his sense of smell. He likes to follow his nose, and he likes to follow and guide me.

When he guides, Fresco shows a similar happiness in his work as Teela does. His head is forward. He has a swift pace and smooth gliding motion to his gait. It is a pleasure walking with him. "It feels natural," I said to the trainer when I first met Fresco to try him out, "natural" having been defined by my past ten years with Teela. As I walked with him on the streets of San Rafael, I looked down and saw, by my side, a golden glow, and I felt as if I were coming home.

Fresco was, like Teela, born in the Guide Dogs kennels. Then he was raised by a family in Fernley, Nevada, near Reno. The father in the family worked as a police officer on an Indian reservation,

243

sometimes assisted by a bomb-sniffing German Shepherd, who was Fresco's companion while growing up. The mother worked at a shelter for abused or neglected children and took Fresco with her. He was patient with the most troubled children. Their daughter taught him to walk quickly while heeling with her, for which I am grateful. According to the family's stories, told to me when I met them at Fresco's guide dog graduation, he carried around a small metal bowl throughout his puppyhood, and he would only sleep on a particular blanket. When the family brought him back to the Guide Dogs campus for his formal training at age fifteen months, they brought his bowl and blanket. "The bowl doesn't have to be metal," the mother told me. "You can get him a plastic one"—the originals having long since disappeared. At present, Fresco has a favorite bed and blanket to the left of where I sit at my desk. He goes to this bed at all times when nothing else is happening. It is, says Hannah, "his home base." He has a tendency to choose the softest dog beds in the house, which has troubled Teela, who has wanted to play with him since the start and whose only condition has been that he not take over her beds.

In place of the bowl, I have given him a white, stuffed fuzzy bone that he carries around, though not continually, and shows to visitors. He likes to take things in his mouth and strut about with them, showing them off. This is different from Teela's habit of retrieving. She wants to retrieve an item and have you toss it to her, while Fresco wants to display that he has it.

He is the "new boy" in our house, the baby, the dog who everyone looks at curiously, wondering what he will do next, what his personality is, how he will evolve with us. For me, he is my excellent guide, my furry friend, my new pair of eyes.

Because of my home and work responsibilities, I was trained with Fresco in the area where I live in San Francisco, rather than on the Guide Dogs campus and the streets of San Rafael, where I trained with Teela. It was an intensive two weeks. I had to learn new techniques, particularly since Fresco was taught to do guide work with the use of food rewards, while Teela was trained to work for praise. During the training, I learned to give him a small piece of his kibble at each curb when he stopped and when he did something good like circling around a garbage can or ignoring a distracting person or dog. At first, it felt wrong to be giving him pieces of food rather than something that felt more natural—a pat on the head or a quick "good dog"—as I had done with Teela. With her, I felt she was stopping at a curb for me, rather than for a treat. But I have grown more accustomed to the new practice over time and through the gradual tapering off of the number of food rewards I give him.

Fresco wears a different style harness than Teela did, a lighter weight leather harness with a less flexible feel to the handle. I missed Teela's harness initially, as I did her, and I wanted the same on him. I wanted him to walk as she did—with a similar bounce in his step— to strain forward at a curb as she did, as if she wished not to stop, then to look back up at me with delight, look around at every crossing not only for traffic but for what might most interest her next. Perhaps there would be a party down the block, a new dog, something to stimulate play.

But Fresco is more businesslike, a more serious dog. He stops on the spot at curbs, turns his nose toward me to see if I will offer him a treat. With Teela, I often felt I took my life in my hands. Would she stop at the curb as she was taught, or would she overstep it and rush on, since moving fast gave us both such enjoyment? "Halt," I would say to her under my breath at each crossing, as if I had to remind her. Fresco stops with a sudden jolt. He races with his swift pace to the curb edge, then puts on the brakes. Sometimes I fear he will overstep a curb so I slow us down as I feel we are getting near it. But we are not there yet. He leads me farther, then halts. I feel more secure with him at curbs. Perhaps he will always pause at them for me. Perhaps he is a better guide dog than Teela. Or I want him to be better to make up for my loss.

It should not have felt like a loss. Here was this new golden dog—a bright orange color, like burnt butterscotch—compared to Teela's more reddish strawberry blond. Here was this mass of furry attentiveness. He was eager to go out, willing to lead, dutiful about getting his treats, loving, putting his nose up to my face for petting. He was fresh life, a younger dog, the new adventure I had wished for. I shouldn't have been so upset, but I was. During those two weeks of the training—on streets, on buses, down on the university campus, in and out of stores—I cried almost every morning before we set out. My tears seemed inexplicable, but, of course, there was an explanation—a big golden girl who now stayed home, but who had been by my side for ten years, sharing every breath, every step, and sharing, most of all, her personality—her glee, her zest, her happiness in life. Early on, I realized that I needed to get a better sense of Fresco—his temperament, his personality, what he liked. So much of my enjoyment of places I had been over the years and, indeed, of my basic experience of life had been filtered through my sense of Teela's enjoyment—how did she feel there, did she want to play Frisbee?

Searching for a better sense of my new guide and of how he took in the world, as soon as my training period was over, I took him one weekend afternoon to the park down the street where Teela always loved to go. I wanted to see how he would respond. We turned right into the gate, walked along the path next to the playing field, where Teela would usually run off in search of a tennis ball to retrieve so I could throw it to her. Yet here I was with a dog who did not retrieve, whose personality was more understated, who dutifully turned right into the park when I asked, then left along the far fence to a place where we sat down on bleachers along with people watching a baseball game played by little children, maybe eight years old. They ran around the bases with much cheering and "good job" called out from the parents and coaches. "Go, go, go," they called in a general air of excitement. I sat there, my new guide dog by my side, and I felt his head turn toward the children out on the field. He was alert. He seemed to enjoy it. He was definitely interested. Perhaps, I later thought, he was looking for one of the boys who had petted him and pulled his hair at the shelter where he went with his raisers during his puppyhood. As I reached down to stroke him, I felt that my new guide was coming alive. I felt happy to be able to share this moment of pleasure and vibrancy with him. I would be okay. I simply had to learn his ways, his interests, what brought him satisfaction, what aroused him. I wanted to go more places with him to find out what it was like to have him as my companion. How did he experience the open-air weekend market I liked to go to? Could I share his particular appreciation of life? "He likes baseball," I said to Hannah when we arrived home, as if that summed it up.

With Teela, her temperament, her personality, her pleasures had been easier for me to find than Fresco's, more on the surface—her constant readiness for play, her quick attentiveness. Fresco's personality was more hidden, more subdued and evenly paced, especially at first. Perhaps it was the discipline of the training, but also the new environment, the city, and coming into our house—a house with two other dogs and three cats—coming into the life of strangers. In the first week of our training, Fresco simply lay down much of the time when he was not working. He would go to a rug on the floor, curl into a ball, and rest. When we were out waiting at a bus stop, he lay down and curled into a ball on the sidewalk. Once in the street in front of our house where I was giving him an opportunity to relieve, confused by the commotion of construction two houses up, he lay down on the asphalt—his answer when things got to be too much, when it was not clear for what purpose he was here. I pulled him up quickly, dismayed. How could I go on with a dog who lay down in the street?

He lay down in buses, as well, when I wanted him to sit. I turned to the trainer, who said to me, "You have to show him what you want. If you want him to sit up in the bus, raise his collar; offer him a piece of food. Prop him up for a while between your legs. He'll get the idea." So again I was bolstering a guide dog between my legs on a bus to hold him upright, though, this time not because his legs were weak, but because this baby dog was out of his element, and when in doubt, when overwhelmed, he retreated to safety.

During the training, beginning the first day, whenever Fresco and I approached another dog on the sidewalk, he stopped. His tail went down between his legs and he would not continue to guide me. The trainer, inquiring, learned that, two weeks earlier, Fresco had been bitten by a Pug on the streets of San Rafael. We had to work with him for many sessions—offering him treats, petting him, reassuring him every time we got near another dog, so it would seem like a wonderful thing, and eventually it did. I was beginning to learn about what my new guide needed, and it worried me. He was a big, strong, male Labrador and the tiniest white Bichon unnerved him. Even the wind at first seemed to scare him. But each challenge, each exposure to something we had to work on, made me want, all the more, for my new guide to succeed. I suddenly did not want to lose him. Perhaps it was the smooth glide to his walk, the way his golden coat shone, the way he reminded me of Teela, the need I had for a guide. As we neared the end of the training period, when the trainer said that Fresco finally was no longer afraid of other dogs—he would be able to guide me safely—and that I was now well prepared to be on my own, I was overjoyed.

Yet there remained much to do. In those weeks of the training and immediately afterward, all of us worked to bring Fresco out of his shell. I asked everyone who came into the house to help me perk him up, get him excited, stimulate him, encourage him to show his happiness in meeting people. Let him know that what was expected of him was life, not deference, not withdrawal. And Teela, as if she knew exactly what was needed, stepped in to help. She got down on the ground on her belly and elbows, rump in the air, and invited him to play. She tried to play with him constantly—attempting, in particular, to teach him how *she* played—how a guide dog, a mature Golden Retriever or Labrador should play. I was amazed at how, from the start, she pawed at Fresco, wanting him to get down on the floor with her. He did not seem to know how to play in the way she wished, so she patiently tried to school him. She would get down on her haunches, open her mouth, and reach up to signal him to come down with her. These two big golden dogs would be standing together—Teela at sixty-eight pounds, Fresco slightly lighter at sixty-one pounds but solid. Teela would put her face up to Fresco's, open her mouth, show him her teeth, take her left front paw and tap at his neck or his shoulder to signal him to get down to the floor so that they could wrestle and roll around mouth to mouth. Teela is so gentle, and Fresco is even more accommodating. They would not hurt each other, but this was guide dog play, or the guide dog play I was used to with Teela, that I had first been exposed to back when she and I were in guide dog school. It is the kind of play she engaged in with her siblings—with her sister Tina, who was also in our training class.

When Teela pawed at Fresco, I knew what she was doing and I rooted for her. He was slow on the uptake, as if he did not quite recognize her style as play. I think he may have wanted to chase her, or to throw himself at her—to interact in some other style. Or he just wanted to sit there and be still in the face of this twelve-year-old, larger dog who gently patted him and insisted that he go down. I watched Teela's efforts and it took nearly a month until Fresco understood, and then he was down and they were mouth to mouth. Their playing with each other has seemed to me more important, at times, than my tie with either dog, though perhaps that is not so. When Hannah, Fresco, and I went on our New Mexico trip two months later, I thought that Fresco would miss Teela, and that Teela would miss Fresco more than she did me. They had become, by then, so intertwined.

Their play reflects their unique bond and, increasingly, it has incorporated Fresco's style. He will take a rubber bone in his mouth, then Teela will grab one end and they will each gently tug. This rubber bone is either orange, blue, or bright green—we have several—and, remarkably, because both dogs are deferential, neither wants to pull the bone entirely out of the other dog's mouth. So they will walk around with it from room to room, each holding one end, stepping in tandem as if hitched, until finally one dog lets the bone go. It's a curious sight, a milling about, these two golden shapes of about the same height, seeming to float in mid-air, holding the bone, jostling each other. Their play seems both an expression of their deferential personalities and of their desires to be close.

With Teela's help and with our human efforts to give Fresco permission to get excited when people came to the house and encouragement to be active, rather than to withdraw, gradually over the first month he stepped out of his shell. He sprung forward happily when the doorbell rang, grabbed his bone and showed it to visitors, elevated when a favorite person arrived. He stopped lying down in buses and on sidewalks, instead began to stand erect and watchful, looking for interest, his nose sniffing the air. Often now when he and I come back from an afternoon of guidework, when we enter the basement where Teela is usually waiting, Fresco races from the front to the back of the long space, flips himself in mid-air, lunges for Teela's shoulder and her neck, runs and flips again. He is letting out his extra energy, bridled when in the harness, becoming free. And Teela is part of it, welcoming him back, nuzzling him, ready to play.

At times, Fresco plays with Teela her way, getting down on the ground, where he rolls over on his back like a puppy deferring to an elder. This is not quite Teela's style, but close. Their mouths open to one another showing teeth as they go for each other's throats. Fresco's more natural style of play is to rise up in the air to wrestle with another dog at the neck, while Teela's is to go down, then wrestle while on her belly. Possibly the difference is because of their different builds. Teela's strength is in her powerful upper chest and front legs; she does not rise on her hind legs easily. Fresco's rear legs are like springs; he enjoys launching himself through the air with them—a missile flying up the stairs, or onto a bed, or at the neck of my golden girl. I think Teela would rather be down on the ground, steadying herself on her haunches or elbows, using her mouth and her front paws. Yet she tolerates Fresco's style, growling as she tries to keep him level as they play and romp like dogs.

In the evening, when Hannah and I sit in our living room, these two big golden dogs lie at our feet—Teela on her bed, Fresco on a new blanket I have lain down for him—and Hannah and I marvel at how lucky we are, how fortunate. How special it is to have the company of two guide dogs, two calm yet responsive beings whose presence is a testament not only to my loss of eyesight, but also to all the work that went into raising and training them.

With three dogs and three cats, it is considerable work for me. I tell myself, over and over, "It's because of my eyesight. You have to do extra when you are blind." One of the costs of getting a guide dog is that you care for it. And now we have two.

"You think you need something outside yourself with exactly Teela's temperament to make you happy," my sister said to me during my training when I was sad. "You can't believe it now, but your happiness doesn't depend on that."

When the trainer arrived for one of our first sessions, I asked him, "Do you think Fresco will ever retrieve?" I was hesitant to ask because this attribute seemed to me beside the point of guidework, not what the trainer was here for, an extra that most people might not even want. But retrieving a floppy Frisbee had been so important in my relationship with Teela. I think the trainer sensed the depth of my desire. He began each session, from then on, by picking up one of Teela's floppy Frisbees as soon as he arrived, getting all excited about it, waving it in the air, making high-pitched, delighted noises, and tossing it to Fresco. Fresco ran after it down the length of the basement, then came back without it. Eventually he did pick it up once or twice and brought it back in our direction, but he quickly lost interest. "It may not be in his nature," the trainer said. We tried giving him food rewards for picking up the Frisbee from the floor and bringing it to me, using a clicker to train his focus on it, but Fresco simply took the food and came to nuzzle for petting, leaving the Frisbee behind. He did not seem to grasp the concept of picking up this piece of watermelon-red cloth that had so thrilled Teela.

I next tried tossing the Frisbee to Teela in Fresco's presence—in the basement, and later at the beach—so that Fresco would see her catching it and bringing it to me, full of joy. He ran after her, but not the Frisbee. He tried grabbing it in his mouth while it was in hers occasionally, tugging at it. They then would both hold it, as they did the bone, in his style of play. But that did not translate into retrieving. I bought a big green plastic Frisbee and offered it to Fresco, thinking plastic might be easier for him to pick up than cloth, or that it would make more sense as something he might retrieve. For I had found that he liked a small yellow plastic Frisbee we had in the house, well chewed on from when our pet poodle, Esperanza, was a puppy. He picked it up and carried it around with great pleasure, as if it was a long-lost friend. But I think that may have been because it reminded him of his bowl. When I tossed him the green plastic Frisbee, he ran toward it enthusiastically at first—as if he recognized it as desirable—then ran past it and began to sniff the ground. Sometimes he pounced on it, picked it up, carried it proudly, then sat down and chewed on it. It was clearly a prize for him, if not an object to be brought back to me. Still, he showed more interest in it than he had in the floppy version.

When I began preparing for our trip to the desert, I packed the green plastic Frisbee carefully in a box along with Fresco's food, feeling hopeful, looking forward to when we would be out in the open and I would throw the Frisbee to him and he would finally retrieve. Playing Frisbee with Teela had always been a way I gave her exercise while we traveled. When in the desert, she and I would go out early in the morning before getting in the car and play a round of "fetch." She would then contentedly climb in for the trip. When I played Frisbee with her during a day, I felt I made her happy. I loved to see her run, blurry and disappearing as her shape might be. I delighted in her broad Golden Retriever smile on bringing the Frisbee back to me. Her joy gave me joy; her motion through the air made me feel I, too, was flying.

My playing Frisbee with her not only gave Teela exercise, but it was a way I kept her from wandering off, following her nose and eating things out of my sight. It was as if she was attached to me by a very long leash—because she would always come back to have me throw to her again. On our trips in the desert, the Frisbee traveled in the back of the SUV, where I put it, often wet from her saliva, to dry out during the day. Teela knew it was there and would stand beside me when I lifted the back car door, alert, nose in the air, eyes tuned, waiting for it to emerge. In all of our travels over the years—when I visited my mother back East, on the days when I taught on the university campus and had extra time, when I attended a conference and had to stay in a motel, anywhere I went, when I needed escape, I would take the Frisbee out of my bag, call Teela to me, and we would go out and play. On our trips to the desert, I always carried two Frisbees with me on the chance that I would toss one accidentally off to a place where neither of us could find it. It was too precious to lose.

When this December, I took the green plastic Frisbee with me—and a floppy backup just in case—and then took it out high in the Pinos Altos hills on the dirt road where Teela once had chased it, I was looking for the same exuberant joy as I had experienced with her—as if Fresco would be freed by the mountain air, as if now he would become my beloved old companion. I waved the Frisbee at him excitedly, tossed it high in the air, but low enough for him to track it. I threw it to him on clear days and in the snow and in mornings when we were fresh. Each time, as I, with great enthusiasm, called his attention to the upcoming throw, he eyed me determinedly, happy to be called into action, waiting, ready, nose in air, body poised. And then he took off, ran in the direction of the toss, then ran right past it—to a spot nearby, where he happily lowered his nose and smelled the very interesting ground.

I then had to walk down the road, fetch the Frisbee, and try again. I was determined. He was obliging, but clearly he had no retriever instinct. Or I like to think he had part of the instinct. He could follow the throw, fly after the prey. He simply did not bring the dead or injured animal back. He had the other end of the drive, as when he would proudly carry around his bone or his fuzzy toy. These had to represent prey. But for him, the lure of the outdoors lay in the scents it offered. The Frisbee led him to new places to explore with his nose. His freedom, his adventure, lay in tracking the smells as Teela's did in chasing her floppy disc.

When Fresco's nose went down and he began to sniff, I would call and call to him out on that desert road, but he would not come to me. I lost sight of him often—his golden shape blending into the blond earth. I lost both my dog and my Frisbee, and part of my deepest dreams, at least for a while—until I spied some movement near bushes in the distance that I could run to. Then I took Fresco by the collar and we both went in search of the green Frisbee. I tried putting a piece of food on top of it when we found it, seeking to teach Fresco to "Find the Frisbee," but this was a search I was dead set on, not one that mattered much to him.

Thus on our trip, I was left getting the exercise I had wished for my guide while Fresco sniffed the snow and earth. It has taken me a while, and I am not yet fully there, to appreciate that Fresco takes as much pleasure from his sense of smell as Teela does from catching an object on the fly, and it is as all-engrossing to him.

WHEN HANNAH AND I WERE TRAVELING in New Mexico for those three weeks, I noticed that I started almost every statement I made about Fresco with a comparison: "Teela would be panting and shedding right now," I'd say as Fresco sat quietly at my feet on the plane and it began to take off. "Teela wouldn't want to get on that bus," I said in the airport when we approached the shuttle that would take us to the rental car agency. "Teela would know the way to the elevator," I noted in the terminal. "Teela would have a hard time jumping up into the rental SUV." "Teela would play Frisbee with me." "Do you remember the time when I forgot Teela's dinner and I had to order her a chicken sandwich in the restaurant?" "Teela always peed more easily than Fresco in unfamiliar places." "Teela would be happy to be here, she liked the desert," or so I hoped. After a while of this constant comparison, in which Fresco often came off as second best, I told Hannah, "I have to stop prefacing every statement I make about Fresco with a comparison to Teela. I have to discipline myself to do that even if it's what I think I want to say."

Soon afterward, I drew up a list of observations about Fresco stated without comparison with Teela—as if I were describing him to someone else. That exercise helped me to see him separately, to appreciate his endearing qualities:

He is sparkling orange in color when seen outside in sunlight. But his color varies with changes in light. Sometimes he looks a lighter tan and, at other times, like dark honey.

He is well built, relatively tall, though slight and sleek for a Lab—a long body, muscular legs. When we are out, people sometimes say, "What a good-looking dog," "What a beautiful dog." Or, "He's pretty."

His puppy raisers told me he was the smartest of the five guide dog puppies they had raised. They called him by the nickname "Bubba."

When I went with him to his veterinary exam during my training, the Guide Dogs veterinarian said he was the "sensitive type."

His eyes look thoughtful. He has extra skin above them that wrinkles thickly sometimes, making him look like a bloodhound, or simply quizzical. I know about his appearance both from what I see and feel, and from what people tell me. Sometimes I will see Fresco more clearly in photographs blown up on my computer screen than I do in real life. His expressions are earnest.

He remembers things. During our training, on our first walk to the local commercial street in my neighborhood, we stopped into a bank to give Fresco practice entering stores. The next time we walked down that block, he took me directly to the bank's front door without instruction. When we were training on the university campus, he followed the broad sweeps of the leash as I indicated a complex route I wanted him to follow—along paths and across main thoroughfares—then remembered the route on coming back. He remembers every corner on which I have ever given him a treat.

His movements, when he guides me, are fluid. As he weaves me around scaffolds and garbage cans, I feel I am being taken for a very smooth ride. Yet at corners, he turns sharply left or right, as instructed, with movements so precise that I feel as if I am in the army. He stops promptly at curbs, although he will try to keep going on the upcurb if he senses I am not coming to a complete stop. He will go as fast as my legs will carry me so that often I am almost running as he guides me. Yet at other times—such as when I hurt my knee and needed to walk down hills slowly—he decreased his pace without instruction, as if he knew to compensate for my limp.

In supermarkets, he guides me carefully in small spaces—turning responsively down narrow aisles, stopping when I do, his pace slower than when outdoors. Though he will also take pride in zooming down the aisles if I wish—as we did on our New Mexico trip when we raced from one end of Walmart to the other. As we whizzed by other customers, I thought I heard them mumble, "What a good-looking dog!"

In stores when I stand handling items, he stands by my side patiently without pulling. He is capable of standing so still when I am taking photographs that the camera does not shake.

One weekend not long after my training, I walked with him to a local outdoor produce market, where I stood handling vegetables. I was surprised that he did not extend his tongue to swipe Brussels sprouts or strawberries from the counter, nor put his nose down to pick up scraps from the ground. After I made my purchases, we went over to a nearby park bench, where I bent down to put my bag of produce in my backpack. I broke off a piece of fresh squash that I had tasted and found sweet and held the piece out to Fresco. He nosed toward it, barely deigning to smell it, then turned away. He would not eat just anything. Later I noticed that the piece was missing from my bag. I felt glad that he had eaten it after all, for I wanted to share my pleasures with him. But two weeks later, I found that piece of squash dried up, deep in the bottom of my pack. He had dutifully taken it in his mouth and dropped it there for me. I like to think it was a measure of his thoughtfulness.

Fresco will occasionally try to eat items on the sly, more now than when he first came to me. But he will usually drop them on command. I think that when his nose is down, he is primarily inhaling for an understanding of his environment, rather than looking for objects to ingest.

When he noses among the plants in our yard, he takes careful steps and stretches his body to explore in all directions, and his graceful movements remind me of those of a cat.

Fresco has not yet mastered the back seats of cars. He slides around on the seat when our car stops suddenly or when it lurches up or down San Francisco hills. When we travel with three dogs, Esperanza and Teela take the back seat, because they are senior, and Fresco gets the floor. Sitting there behind Hannah, he stretches his nose forward over the center console between the two front seats and nuzzles me.

He loves expressions of affection. He has a gentle way of putting his head in my lap for petting.

He lets me brush his teeth right after his dinner each night—needed to keep his plaque under control—and he reminds me when I forget. He sits on the rug waiting.

Sometimes he jumps up on beds. The first time I found him on our bed, I snuck away to get my camera, took his picture, then instructed him sternly to get down.

I think he has a stubborn streak, as when I call him while he is sniffing and he will not come. But usually when I call his name or whistle, he races toward me.

He pees by squatting, not by lifting his leg, and it's always clear when he is doing this since the sound is strong.

He doesn't drink a lot.

When he lies down to rest or sleep, he almost always curls in a ball.

He follows me. He likes to be near me.

He likes lying close to Teela, and he loves to play with her. Some mornings, playing with her is the first thing he does.

When Fresco, Hannah, and I returned from our trip to the desert, Fresco and Teela went nose to nose, sniffing each other, getting reacquainted. Then they settled down, lying near each other in the kitchen. It was a quiet homecoming, all of us back where we belonged, back with our pack. It had been an unusual trip for me—a new opening, a reminder of what I had yet to do. I had yet to learn how to accept my new guide fully, how to make my peace with the fact that he was not Teela, how to enjoy him and trust him. As we settled in at home, I went back to work at my computer, Fresco on his bed by my side, Teela across the room on her bed, the cats on my desk and file cabinet, Esperanza coming in and out. I looked at my pictures taken while on our trip. There was Fresco in the snow, his muzzle covered with white. He had eaten the snow whenever he could and put his nose down through it to smell the earth below. He had not run in it, but probed it. He had done his Fresco thing—enraptured, hard to pull away. There he was—burnt butterscotch against the white, against the golden tan dirt of the desert, or on a blanket I had lain down next to the table where I sat loading my pictures into my iPad. He was taking his place by my side in the same position as he had adopted when back at home.

Then two weeks after our return, one morning when Fresco and Teela were playing in the living room in the sunlight, I noticed that Teela, standing over Fresco, was licking his neck. He lay like a puppy rolled on his back, mouth open toward her, not appearing to mind. But it soon seemed to me she was licking him obsessively, so much so that I told her to stop. I did not want her rubbing his skin raw. She stopped. They kept playing. Late that day, they played again—in the room downstairs in our basement. Again, I noticed that Teela was licking Fresco's neck, and I asked her to stop.

The following morning after he woke, when I touched Fresco's neck before attaching his leash, I felt a stickinesss on his upper chest just below his neck. I took him out to relieve; then, before his breakfast, I took a washcloth and thoroughly washed the area to remove the stickiness. I used soap, rinsed, then felt again—still sticky. It was blood. That is what Teela had been licking, cleaning him before I did. I applied antiseptic and we took Fresco to the vet.

The vet could not find evidence of puncture wounds, but the spots where two welts had risen on Fresco's chest seemed to me like places where Teela's teeth once had been. Perhaps she bit him accidentally in play. Perhaps her teeth had simply grazed him there.

Probably my subsequent use of the collar and harness, while he guided me, further aggravated the wound. Maybe his sores—covering an area of several inches square and visible when the veterinarian cut away Fresco's hair to treat them—were caused by something other than Teela's teeth. Perhaps the harness itself had done this, or something caught beneath it had rubbed Fresco's upper chest raw. Whatever the case, my new guide dog was injured. My old guide dog may have been at fault. But I felt I was at fault—because I had not noticed. Of course, I could not see the wound, could not see a bite or an abrasion, or the color of blood. But I had thought that the stickiness was candy, or a substance that Fresco had picked up from plants in the yard. Blood did not occur to me at first, because my guide dog was not one to be injured. He was safe, pure, young, new, mine, unscathed.

The veterinarian gave me an ointment to apply to Fresco's wounds twice a day and medicine to give him twice a day that would decrease the inflammation. The medicine made Fresco woozy. The ointment was oily. I couldn't walk with him for almost a week, because I did not want his collar or harness to rub on the area of his sores and further inflame them. During that time, I felt the loss of my new guide. I felt his vulnerability. Every morning and every evening, as I applied the ointment, rubbing it with my fingers into his sores—even as they became less inflamed—I felt in touch with him as I had not before, in a deeper way, more inextricably bound. I could not walk without him. I did not want to go out and do my errands with a cane, go to appointments with my cane. Where before, I had noticed how much Teela and Fresco were interrelated, now I noticed my own bond.

Something changed for me during that week. I took Fresco off the medication early, not liking him doped up. If I was losing my physical guide, I did not want to lose his spirit as well. For by then, he seemed to have a spirit I knew, his "Fresconess." He was not a retriever, not Teela's lively self, not a big white head in my lap, but a darker one. The tides had shifted, and the new boy—the replacement—was now the one on whose life I depended, as he did on mine. This is not to say that I lost my vital connection with Teela. Our bond is strong, her presence is with me every day, so much so that I still have to make sure that it does not overshadow Fresco's.

"I have two guide dogs," I say to myself at times—as I did a few weeks ago when Hannah, Fresco, Teela, Esperanza, and I were at the beach. It was a calm, sunny day, the waves breaking in the background. Leaving Fresco's harness behind, I took two nylon leashes, attached one to Fresco, and one to Teela, and followed as they guided me along the shore. The leashes, deep royal blue, were hard to distinguish from one another as I sought to keep them from tangling together, just as the dogs were sometimes indistinguishable. They pulled me, but not too strongly. They wanted to go along the cliffs by the shore, to smell, and, for Teela, to lick at the cliffs' edge, where the dampness in the sand catches scents of seaweed and sea birds and dead fish. Teela was leading, I think, more than Fresco, teaching him how to walk with your person along the beach. "Don't dawdle. Keep on sniffing," she said. "Keep on moving, Fresco. You can grab something small to eat, but don't let her see you." They pulled, and she led, and I followed along. "I have two guide dogs," I said to myself, as if it opened up a mystery. I have been that fortunate. I am learning from them about my connections, my relationships—about not replacing one with another, about coming to know each on their own terms.

I am older now than when I first walked with Teela. I have had more richness of experience. Yet I still need to learn, to grow. Each dog has stretched me, made me younger, made me feel more like a dog at times. Each helps me to experience the world more simply, more in terms of pleasures, comforts, and rewards.

At night now as I reach down next to our bed and touch Fresco, I finger his nylon collar—which helps me distinguish him from Teela—"Goodnight. Good guide. Thank you," I say to him. And the words seem strange and new, as if I should not be saying these to any other dog than Teela. Teela comes into the bedroom later. I hear the tinkling of her collar as she enters and gets onto her bed beside Fresco's—a small space dividing them. She lies down. I reach over to touch her, pat her soft fur. "Thank you. Good guide, girl." My tears are slow and gentle. For the moment, I have the company of these two. I will treasure this moment as long as I have it, as long as their two tongues lick me in the morning, their noses wet, fresh from their night's sleep—letting me know they are ready for me, their person— their woman in need of a guide dog—to get up and take them out.

On Teela's neck on her silver collar, I have left the tag that says "guide dog," rather than substituting one that says "retired guide" that Guide Dogs sent me over a year ago. I want Teela never to be retired, but to continue to lead the way for me, even as I follow Fresco. I look to her to help me with him, to help me know what might be possible—that the bond can grow, the depth of feeling be sustained, the learning be unexpected and enjoyed. As I walk with my new guide, I see less than I did when I walked with Teela, for my eyesight has diminished over time, although my life has not diminished but grown. As Fresco pulls me forward, guiding me in his way—prompt turns, a gliding motion to his step, showing me the importance of exploring while sniffing—as I follow this dog who curls into a ball when at home, his body so characteristically his own, as I learn to love him as I did Teela, I hope to be as deserving—of his love, his loyalty, hers as well—as they take me not only along streets but into a world of their pleasures.

At Fresco's graduation ceremony—held on the Guide Dogs campus at the end of our training period—that afternoon out in the sun, the puppy raisers handed their dogs over to their new persons on a broad stage before families and friends. Hannah sat in the audience looking up proudly at Fresco and me. When it came our turn,

I was led across the stage to stand beside the mother of the family who had raised Fresco, with whom he had been sitting. She took his leash and handed him to me, tearfully wishing us well. She and her husband each gave me a warm hug. She then read a statement by their high-school age daughter, who was unable to attend:

> *I once wondered what it would be like to be blind. Although as a little girl I tested this wonderment through the basic blind-fold, I never truly experienced what it was like. Some may say that the God-given gift of sight is man's most important sense, but I with my sight, beg to differ. It has been a definitive fact in every science textbook that there are five senses: taste, smell, sight, touch, and the ability to hear. Through the processes of raising guide dogs, I have discovered a sixth . . . love. . . . The trust that a blind person has for their dog is remarkable. Not only do they trust this dog to not poop in the house, but also to be their eyes. These dogs cross streets, hop onto buses, and go everywhere else in between. . . . I have a strong belief that love surpasses sight in every aspect, and that a guide dog is the epitome of love. Fresco, as you continue on your journey as a guide dog, I wish you the best of everything: the best belly rubs, walks, food, and potty breaks. Good job, Bubba!*

As I walk now with Fresco, with memories of Teela echoing in my mind, I cherish the spirit of those who raised him, the love that went into him, the journey we are on—a longer one than I ever expected. Teela is at home when I am out with Fresco, yet at other times, I walk with her, using my white cane and a leash, or letting her roam free as we go. I play with her, throw her balls and Frisbees to retrieve—our old habits sustaining us, the new ones evolving. And when I am following Fresco, I often hear Teela in my mind talking to us: "I said I would help you. Now, Fresco, remember. Remember to watch out for cars and curbs and holes in the ground where she might trip. Remember that she does not easily trust. Play with her. Retrieve a little. Make it a good life for her. I am turning her over to you now. Keep your paws clean and your heart pure. Fresco, come walk beside me. Come, take her from me." And Fresco lifts his head and turns toward me. "Come," he says. "Come, let me guide you."

February–March 2014

Bibliographic Notes

Bibliographic Notes

HUMAN-ANIMAL STUDIES

NOTABLE OVERVIEWS AND EDITED COLLECTIONS in human-animal studies that provide context for *Come, Let Me Guide You* include: Arnold Arluke and Clinton Sanders, *Between the Species: A Reader in Human-Animal Relationships* (San Francisco: Pearson, 2008); Christopher Blazina, Güler Boyraz, and David Shen-Miller, eds., *The Psychology of the Human-Animal Bond: A Resource for Clinicians and Researchers* (New York: Springer, 2011); Margo DeMello, *Animals and Society: An Introduction to Human-Animal Studies* (New York: Columbia University Press, 2012); Margo DeMello, ed., *Teaching the Animal: Human-Animal Studies across the Disciplines* (Herndon, VA: Lantern Books, 2010); Clifton P. Flynn, ed., *Social Creatures: A Human and Animal Studies Reader* (Herndon, VA: Lantern Books, 2008); Aaron S. Gross and Anne Vallely, eds., *Animals and the Human Imagination: A Companion to Animal Studies* (New York: Columbia University Press, 2012); Samantha Hurn, *Humans and Other Animals: Cross-Cultural Perspectives on Human-Animal Interactions* (London: Pluto Press, 2012); Linda Kalof and Amy Fitzgerald, eds., *The Animals Reader: The Essential Classic and Contemporary Writings* (New York: Bloomsbury Academic, 2007); and Claire Jean Kim and Carla Freccero, eds., "Special Issue on Species/Race/Sex," *American Quarterly* 65, no. 3 (2013).

See also: John Knight, ed., *Animals in Person: Cultural Perspectives on Human-Animal Intimacies* (New York: Bloomsbury Academic, 2005); Robert Lurz, ed., *The Philosophy of Animal Minds* (Cambridge and New York: Cambridge University Press, 2009); Emily Plec, ed., *Perspectives on Human-Animal Communication: Internatural Communication* (New York: Routledge, 2012); Clinton Sanders, *Understanding Dogs* (Philadelphia: Temple University Press, 1999); James Serpell, *In the Company of Animals: A Study of Human-Animal Relationships* (Cambridge and New York: Cambridge University Press, 1996); Julie A. Smith and Robert W. Mitchell, eds., *Experiencing Animal Minds: An Anthology of Animal-Human Encounters* (New York: Columbia University Press, 2012); Paul Waldau, *Animal Studies: An Introduction* (Oxford and New York: Oxford University Press, 2013); and Kari Weil, *Thinking Animals: Why Animal Studies Now?* (New York: Columbia University Press, 2012).

Important prior university press books addressing the guide dog-human experience are: Beth Finke, *Long Time, No See* (Champaign: University of Illinois Press, 2003); and Rod Michalko, *The Two-in-One: Walking with Smokie, Walking with Blindness* (Philadelphia: Temple University Press, 1998). See also: Stephen Kuusisto, *Planet of the Blind* (New York: Delta, 1998).

Histories of guide dog organizations that illumine their mission and the guide dog-human experience include: Miriam Ascarelli, *Independent Vision: Dorothy Harrison Eustis and the Story of The Seeing Eye* (West Lafayette, IN: Purdue University Press, 2010); Fidelco Guide Dog Foundation and Gerri Hirshey, *Trust the Dog: Rebuilding Lives Through Teamwork with Man's Best Friend* (New York: Viking, 2010); and Patrick S. Halley, *Guide Dogs of America: A History* (North Charleston, SC: CreateSpace Independent Publishing, 2012).

For recent popular accounts of guide dog-human relationships, see: Claire Anderson and June Brasgalla, *Sightless in Seattle: Adventures with My Guide Dog* (Charleston, SC: CreateSpace Independent

Publishing, 2012); Lloyd Burlingame, *Two Seeing Eye Dogs Take Manhattan: A Love Story* (Charleston, SC: CreateSpace Independent Publishing, 2012); Mark Carlson, *Confessions of a Guide Dog: The Blonde Leading the Blind* (Bloomington, IN: iUniverse, 2011); Carolyn Wing Greenlee, *Steady Hedy: A Journey through Blindness & Guide Dog School* (Kelseyville, CA: Earthen Vessel Productions, 2010); Michael Hingson and Susy Flory, *Thunder Dog: The True Story of a Blind Man, His Guide Dog, and the Triumph of Trust at Ground Zero* (Nashville, TN: Thomas Nelson, 2011); Julie L. Johnson, *Courage to Dare: A Blind Woman's Quest to Train Her Own Guide Dog* (Amazon Digital Services, 2014); Matthew VanFossan, *Through Gilly's Eyes: Memoirs of a Guide Dog* (Pittsburgh, PA: Volant Press, 2013); and John Edward White, *Dog Lessons: How Raising a Guide Dog Taught Me to See* (Altadena, CA: TeamGruden Publishing, 2012). See also two classics: Bill Irwin and David McCasland, *Blind Courage: A 2,000 Mile Journey of Faith* (Harpers Ferry, WV: Appalachian Trail Conference, 1991); and Betty White and Tom Sullivan, *The Leading Lady: Dinah's Story* (New York: Bantam, 1992).

The benefits of service dog partnerships are discussed in the popular literature in: Kyla Duffy and Lowrey Mumford, *Partners With Paws: Service Dogs and the Lives They Change* (Boulder, CO: Happy Tails Books, 2011); Jane Miller, *Healing Companions: Ordinary Dogs and Their Extraordinary Power to Transform Lives* (Pompton Plains, NJ: New Page Books, 2009); and Kathy Nimmer, *Two Plus Four Equals One: Celebrating the Partnership of People with Disabilities and Their Assistance Dogs* (Indianapolis: Dog Ear Publishing, 2010).

Further general interest works with valuable perspectives on dog-human communication and intimacy are: Brenda Aloff, *Canine Body Language: A Photographic Guide Interpreting the Native Language of the Domestic Dog* (Wenatchee, WA: Dogwise Publishing, 2005); Dawn Baumann Brunke, *Animal Voices, Animal Guides: Discover Your Deeper Self through Communication with Animals* (Rochester, VT: Bear

& Company; 2009); Stanley Coren, *How To Speak Dog: Mastering the Art of Dog-Human Communication* (New York: Atria Books, Simon and Schuster, 2001) and *How Dogs Think: What the World Looks Like to Them and Why They Act the Way They Do* (New York: Atria Books, Simon and Schuster, 2005); David Grimm, *Citizen Canine: Our Evolving Relationship with Cats and Dogs* (New York: PublicAffairs Books: 2014); Donna Haraway, *The Companion Species Manifesto: Dogs, People, and Significant Otherness* (Chicago: Prickly Paradigm Press, 2003); Alexandra Horowitz, *Inside of a Dog: What Dogs See, Smell, and Know* (New York: Scribner, 2010); Patricia B. McConnell, *For the Love of a Dog: Understanding Emotion in You and Your Best Friend* (New York: Ballantine, 2006); David Tabatsky, ed., and Gary Gross, *Beautiful Old Dogs: A Loving Tribute to Our Senior Best Friends* (New York: St. Martin's Press, 2013); and Gene Weingarten and Michael S. Williamson, *Old Dogs: Are the Best Dogs* (New York: Simon and Schuster, 2008).

Notable discussions of animal emotion, cognition, and communication more broadly appear in: Marc Bekoff, *The Emotional Lives of Animals: A Leading Scientist Explores Animal Joy, Sorrow, and Empathy—and Why They Matter* (Novato, CA: New World Library, 2008) and *Why Dogs Hump and Bees Get Depressed: The Fascinating Science of Animal Intelligence, Emotions, Friendship, and Conservation* (Novato, CA: New World Library, 2013); Richard Bulliet, *Hunters, Herders, and Hamburgers: The Past and Future of Human-Animal Relationships* (New York: Columbia University Press, 2007); Margo deMello, ed., *Speaking for Animals: Animal Autobiographical Writing* (New York: Routledge, 2012); Temple Grandin and Catherine Johnson, *Animals in Translation: Using the Mysteries of Autism to Decode Animal Behavior* (New York: Harcourt, 2006); Jeffrey Moussaieff Masson and Susan McCarthy, *When Elephants Weep: The Emotional Lives of Animals* (New York: Delta, 1996); and Jeffrey Moussaieff Masson, *Dogs Never Lie About Love: Reflections on the Emotional World of Dogs* (New York: Broadway Books, 1998).

Critical overviews concerned with animal welfare issues include: Josephine Donovan and Carol Adams, eds., *The Feminist Care Tradition in Animal Ethics* (New York: Columbia University Press, 2007); Lisa A. Kemmerer, ed., *Sister Species: Women, Animals, and Social Justice* (Champaign: University of Illinois Press, 2011); Anthony J. Nocella II, John Sorenson, Kim Socha, and Atsuko Matsuoka, eds., *Defining Critical Animal Studies: An Intersectional Social Justice Approach for Liberation* (New York: Peter Lang International Academic Publishers, 2013); and Wayne Pacelle, *The Bond: Our Kinship with Animals, Our Call to Defend Them* (New York: William Morrow, 2011).

INTIMATE ETHNOGRAPHIC METHOD

The intimate ethnographic approach used in *Come, Let Me Guide You* extends that of my prior studies: *Traveling Blind: Adventures in Vision with a Guide Dog by My Side* (West Lafayette, IN: Purdue University Press, 2010); *Things No Longer There: A Memoir of Losing Sight and Finding Vision* (Madison: University of Wisconsin Press, 2005); *The Family Silver: Essays on Relationships among Women* (Berkeley and Los Angeles: University of California Press, 1996); *Social Science and the Self: Personal Essays on an Art Form* (New Brunswick, NJ: Rutgers University Press, 1991); *The Mirror Dance: Identity in a Women's Community* (Philadelphia: Temple University Press, 1983); and *Hip Capitalism* (Beverly Hills: Sage Publications, 1979).

The quotations used in Chapter 12 are from the above works as follows: from *The Mirror Dance*: "clearly an experiment," page xvii; "multiple-person stream of consciousness," page 187; from *Social Science and the Self*: "I knew I would have to 'assert myself,'" page 182; "We see others as we know ourselves," page 182; from *The Family Silver*: "The intimacy of the essays is their central challenge," page 2; "the easy answers disappear," page 1; "people who know me, for instance, think I look like myself," page 31; from *Things No Longer There*: "She took my hand," page 158; "moving on and growing older," page 1; "a counterposing internal vision," page 93; from *Traveling Blind*: "Like the desert that gradually reclaims," page 8; "the comfort I viewed in the landscape," page 161; "Airports—they are so very public," page 128; and from *Come, Let Me Guide You* (West Lafayette, IN: Purdue University Press, 2015): "In that moment, and in others like it," pages 196–97.

The "turning point" methodological article discussed in Chapter 12 is: "Beyond 'Subjectivity': The Use of the Self in Social Science," *Qualitative Sociology* 8, no. 4 (1985): 309–24 and is included in *Social Science and the Self*: 165–83. I discuss my mixing of genres in *Hip Capitalism* and *The Mirror Dance* in "Fiction and Social Science," *Studies in Symbolic Interaction* 5 (1984): 269–86, reprinted in *The Mirror Dance* as an Appendix: 173–99. In "Research and the Construction of a Text," *Studies in Symbolic Interaction* 2 (1979): 167–87, I discuss the "novelistic" approach of *Hip Capitalism*. I reconsider the multivoiced approach of *The Mirror Dance* in "*The Mirror Dance* Revisited," *Journal of Lesbian Studies* 9, no. 1-2 (2005): 1–9.

My early published personal writings referred to in Chapters 11 and 12 include: "A Trip to the Anza Borrego Desert," *Conditions: One* 1, no. 1: 82–89; "Change," *Conditions: Four* 2, no. 1 (1979): 55–61; and "Ambivalence," *Sinister Wisdom* 8, Winter 1979: 33–37. "Becoming a Lesbian" appears in *The Family Silver*, pages 82–106, excerpted from my unpublished novel, "Jenny's World" (1983).

The quotation from *Traveling Blind* in Chapter 13, "We had a good dinner that night back up in Silver City," appears in that book on pages 48–49.

Further helpful discussions of the use of self-reflection in ethnography can be found in: Tony E. Adams, Stacy Holman Jones, and Carolyn Ellis, *Autoethnography* (New York: Oxford University Press, 2015); Robin M. Boylorn and Mark P. Orbe, eds.,

Critical Autoethnography: Intersecting Cultural Identities in Everyday Life (Walnut Creek, CA: Left Coast Press, 2013); Peter Collins and Anselma Gallinat, eds., *The Ethnographic Self As Resource: Writing Memory and Experience into Ethnography* (Oxford and New York: Berghahn Books, 2010); and Stacy Holman Jones, Tony E. Adams, and Carolyn Ellis, eds., *Handbook of Autoethnography* (Walnut Creek, CA: Left Coast Press, 2013). Feminist methodologies are explored in: Sharlene Nagy Hesse-Biber, ed., *Handbook of Feminist Research: Theory and Praxis*, Second Edition (Thousand Oaks, CA: Sage Publications, 2011) and *Feminist Research Practice: A Primer*, Second Edition (Thousand Oaks, CA: Sage Publications, 2013). See also: Christa Craven and Dána-Ain Davis, eds., *Feminist Activist Ethnography: Counterpoints to Neoliberalism in North America* (New York: Lexington Books, 2013); Carolyn Ellis, "Telling Secrets, Revealing Lives: Relational Ethics in Research with Intimate Others," *Qualitative Inquiry* 13, no. 1 (2007): 3–29 and *Revision: Autoethnographic Reflections on Life and Work* (Walnut Creek, CA: Left Coast Press, 2008); and Mary Jo Maynes, Jennifer L. Pierce, and Barbara Laslett, *Telling Stories: The Use of Personal Narratives in the Social Sciences and History* (Ithaca: Cornell University Press, 2008). Two valuable discussions of truth-seeking objectives in personal and fiction writing that I have found particularly helpful are: Judith Barrington, *Writing the Memoir: From Truth to Art*, Second Edition (Portland, OR: Eighth Mountain Press, 2002); and Ann Patchett, *This is the Story of a Happy Marriage* (New York: Harper, 2013).

WOMEN AND DISABILITIES

THE WOMEN AND DISABILITIES course discussed in Chapter 13 draws from a rich literature on women's experiences that I have gratefully explored each year. The works I used in the course in 2011 are as follows, listed alphabetically by author: Sally Hobart Alexander, *Do You Remember the Color Blue? And Other Questions Kids Ask about Blindness* (New York: Viking, 2000); Amanda Baggs, "Up in the Clouds and Down in the Valley: My Richness and Yours," *Disability Studies Quarterly* 30, no. 1 (2010), http://www.dsq-sds.org/article/view/1052/1238; Ruth Bendor, "Arthritis and I," *Annals of Internal Medicine* 131, no. 2 (1999): 150–52; Brenda Jo Brueggemann, "Interpreting Women," in Bonnie G. Smith and Beth Hutchison, eds., *Gendering Disability* (New Brunswick, NJ: Rutgers University Press, 2004), 61–72; Susan Cahn, "Come Out, Come Out Whatever You've Got! or, Still Crazy after All These Years," *Feminist Studies* 29, no. 1 (2003): 7–18; Sucheng Chan, "You're Short, Besides!," in Asian Women United of California, ed., *Making Waves: An Anthology of Writings by and about Asian American Women* (Boston: Beacon, 1989), 265–73; Eli Clare, "Flirting With You: Some Notes on Isolation and Connection," in Victoria A. Brownworth and Susan Raffo, eds., *Restricted Access: Lesbians on Disability* (Seattle, WA: Seal Press, 1999), 127–35; Vicky D'aoust, "Complications: The Deaf Community, Disability and Being a Lesbian Mom—A Conversation with Myself," in Victoria A. Brownworth and Susan Raffo, eds., *Restricted Access: Lesbians on Disability* (Seattle, WA: Seal Press, 1999), 115–23; Melissa J. Frame, "What's Wrong With Her? The Stigmatizing Effects of an Invisible Stigma," *Disability Studies Quarterly* 20, no. 3 (2000): 243–53; and Beth Finke, *Long Time, No See* (Champaign: University of Illinois Press, 2003).

See also: Mary Felstiner, "Casing My Joints: A Private and Public Story of Arthritis," *Feminist Studies* 24, no. 4 (2000): 273–85 and *Out of Joint: A Private and Public Story of Arthritis* (Lincoln: University of Nebraska Press, 2005); Carolyn Gage, "Hidden Disability: A Coming Out Story," in Victoria A. Brownworth and Susan Raffo, eds., *Restricted Access: Lesbians on Disability* (Seattle, WA: Seal Press, 1999), 201–11; Terry Galloway, "I'm Listening as Hard as I Can," in

Marsha Saxton and Florence Howe, eds., *With Wings: An Anthology of Literature by and about Women with Disabilities* (New York: Feminist Press, 1987), 5–9; Rosemarie Garland-Thomson, "Feminist Disability Studies," *Signs: Journal of Women in Culture and Society* 30, no. 2 (2005): 1557–87; Eileen Garvin, *How to Be a Sister: A Love Story with a Twist of Autism* (New York: The Experiment, 2010); Nadine Goranson, "Silent Trespass," in Peggy Munson, ed., *Stricken: Voices from the Hidden Epidemic of Chronic Fatigue Syndrome* (New York: The Haworth Press, 2000), 53–60; Temple Grandin, *The Way I See It: A Personal Look at Autism and Asperger's* (Arlington, TX: Future Horizons, 2008); Amanda Hamilton, "Oh the Joys of Invisibility," *Electric Edge*, July–August 1997, http://www.ragged-edge -mag.com/archive/look.htm; and Daphne L. Hill, "and I will have sex again," in Shelley Tremain, ed., *Pushing the Limits: Disabled Dykes Produce Culture* (Ontario, Canada: Women's Press, 1996), 72–76.

Further personal accounts discussed include: Harriet McBryde Johnson, *Too Late to Die Young: Nearly True Tales from a Life* (New York: Henry Holt, 2005); Kay Redfield Jamison, *An Unquiet Mind: A Memoir of Moods and Madness* (New York: Vintage, 1997); Megan Jones, "'Gee, You Don't Look Handicapped . . .': Why I Use a White Cane to Tell People that I'm Deaf," *Electric Edge*, July–August 1997, http://www.ragged-edge-mag.com/archive/look.htm; Georgina Kleege, *Sight Unseen* (New Haven: Yale University Press, 1999); Susan Krieger, *Traveling Blind: Adventures in Vision with a Guide Dog by My Side* (West Lafayette, IN: Purdue University Press, 2010), *Traveling Blind: Adventures in Vision with a Guide Dog by My Side,* narrated by Ann M. Richardson (Hertford, NC.: Crossroad Press, 2011), Audible edition, and "The Passing Down of Sorrow," in *The Family Silver: Essays on Relationships among Women* (Berkeley and Los Angeles: University of California Press, 1996), 82–106; Nomy Lamm, "Private Dancer: Evolution of a Freak," in Victoria A. Brownworth and Susan Raffo, eds., *Restricted Access: Lesbians on Disability* (Seattle, WA: Seal

Press, 1999), 152–61; and Simi Linton, *My Body Politic: A Memoir* (Ann Arbor: University of Michigan Press, 2006).

See also: Audre Lorde, *The Cancer Journals* (San Francisco: Spinsters Ink, 1980); Nancy Mairs, *Waist-High in the World: A Life among the Nondisabled* (Boston: Beacon, 1996) and "On Living Behind Bars," in *Plaintext: Deciphering a Woman's Life* (New York: Harper and Row, 1986): 125-54; Martha Manning, "The Legacy," in Nell Casey, ed., *Unholy Ghost: Writers on Depression* (New York: Morrow, 2001); Lorna Moorhead, *Coffee in the Cereal: The First Year with Multiple Sclerosis* (Oxnard, CA: Pathfinder Publishing, 2003) and *Phone in the Fridge: Five Years with Multiple Sclerosis* (Tucson: Pathfinder Publishing, 2006); Judith Moses, "Connections," in Shelley Tremain, ed., *Pushing the Limits: Disabled Dykes Produce Culture* (Ontario, Canada: Women's Press, 1996), 204–5; Christine Miserandino, "The Spoon Theory," (2003), http://www.butyoudontlooksick .com/wpress/articles/written-by-christine/the-spoon-theory; Frances Lief Neer, *Dancing in the Dark* (San Francisco, CA: Wildstar Publishing, 1994); Joan Nestle, "When Tiredness Gives Way to Tiredness," in Peggy Munson, ed., *Stricken: Voices from the Hidden Epidemic of Chronic Fatigue Syndrome* (New York: The Haworth Press, 2000), 39–42; and Margaret A. Nosek et al., "The Meaning of Health for Women with Physical Disabilities: A Qualitative Analysis," *Family & Community Health* 27, no. 1 (2004): 6–21.

Additional valuable narratives are: Deborah Peifer, "Seeing is Be(liev)ing" in Victoria A. Brownworth and Susan Raffo, eds., *Restricted Access: Lesbians on Disability* (Seattle, WA: Seal Press, 1999), 31–34; Mary Frances Platt, "Passing through Shame" and "Personal Assistance," in Victoria A. Brownworth and Susan Raffo, eds., *Restricted Access: Lesbians on Disability* (Seattle, WA: Seal Press, 1999), 180–91; Jen Robinson, "Invisible Illnesses, Visible Stereotypes," in "Sick Chicks and Twisted Sisters: Empowering Disabled Women on the Web," originally at http://sickchicks.homestead

.com/invisibleillness.htm (Fall 2000) and "Homeless While Disabled with a Chronic Illness," originally at http://www.womensstudies .homestead.com (2000); Joan Tollifson, "Imperfection is a Beautiful Thing: On Disability and Meditation," in Kenny Fries, ed., *Staring Back: The Disability Experience from the Inside Out* (New York: Plume/Penguin, 1997), 105–12; Sharon Wachsler, "Still Femme," in Victoria A. Brownworth and Susan Raffo, eds., *Restricted Access: Lesbians on Disability* (Seattle, WA: Seal Press, 1999), 109–14; Alice Walker, "Beauty: When the Other Dancer Is the Self," in Marsha Saxton and Florence Howe, eds., *With Wings: An Anthology of Literature by and about Women with Disabilities,* (New York: Feminist Press, 1987), 152–58; Dorothy Wall, "Encounters with the Invisible," in Peggy Munson, ed., *Stricken: Voices from the Hidden Epidemic of Chronic Fatigue Syndrome* (New York: The Haworth Press, 2000), 23–30; Susan Wendell, *The Rejected Body: Feminist Philosophical Reflections on Disability* (New York: Routledge, 1996); and Patricia Nell Warren, "Autoimmune Disease: A Personal Perspective," in Victoria A. Brownworth and Susan Raffo, eds., *Restricted Access: Lesbians on Disability* (Seattle, WA: Seal Press, 1999), 81–89.

For further helpful recent discussions, see: Katherine Bouton, *Shouting Won't Help: Why I—and 50 Million Other Americans—Can't Hear You* (New York: Sarah Crichton Books/Farrar, Straus and Giroux, 2013); Lennard J. Davis, ed., *The Disability Studies Reader*, Fourth Edition (New York: Routledge, 2013); Kim Q. Hall, ed., *Feminist Disability Studies* (Bloomington: Indiana University Press, 2011); Alison Kafer, *Feminist, Queer, Crip* (Bloomington: Indiana University Press, 2013); Nicole C. Kear, *Now I See You: A Memoir* (New York: St. Martin's Press, 2014); Heather Kuttai, *Maternity Rolls: Pregnancy, Childbirth and Disability* (Halifax and Winnipeg, Canada: Fernwood Publishing, 2010); Cynthia Lewiecki-Wilson and Jen Cellio, eds., *Disability and Mothering: Liminal Spaces of Embodied Knowledge* (Syracuse: Syracuse University Press, 2011); Susannah B. Mintz, *Unruly*

Bodies: Life Writing by Women with Disabilities (Chapel Hill: University of North Carolina Press, 2007); Harilyn Rousso, *Don't Call Me Inspirational: A Disabled Feminist Talks Back* (Philadelphia: Temple University Press, 2013); Laurie Rubin, *Do You Dream in Color?: Insights from a Girl without Sight* (New York: Seven Stories Press, 2012); Elyn R. Saks, *The Center Cannot Hold: My Journey Through Madness* (New York: Hyperion, 2007); Ellen Samuels, *Fantasies of Identification: Disability, Gender, Race* (New York and London: New York University Press, 2014); Sonia Sotomayor, *My Beloved World: A Memoir* (New York: Knopf, 2012); and Caitlin Wood, ed., *Criptiques* (Portland, OR: May Day, 2014).